WHO LIVES, WHO DIES
WITH KIDNEY DISEASE

MOHAMMAD AKMAL AND
VASUNDHARA RAGHAVAN

Who Lives, Who Dies with Kidney Disease

iUniverse books may be ordered through booksellers or by contacting:

iUniverse
1663 Liberty Drive
Bloomington, IN 47403
www.iuniverse.com
1-800-Authors (1-800-288-4677)

Because of the dynamic nature of the Internet, any web addresses or links contained in this book may have changed since publication and may no longer be valid. The views expressed in this work are solely those of the author and do not necessarily reflect the views of the publisher, and the publisher hereby disclaims any responsibility for them.

Any people depicted in stock imagery provided by Getty Images are models, and such images are being used for illustrative purposes only.
Certain stock imagery © Getty Images.

ISBN: 978-1-5320-4846-3 (sc)
ISBN: 978-1-5320-4847-0 (e)

Library of Congress Control Number: 2018905951

Print information available on the last page.

iUniverse rev. date: 06/14/2018

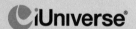

Contents

The most important thing in illness is never to lose heart.
—Nikolai Lenin

Introduction

Dealing with illness, particularly major diseases, has always been a challenge. How an illness affects a person is determined by factors such as physical condition, family circumstance, economic background, and personal attitude. Patients relying heavily on medical experts' advice find it easier to manage the disease, whereas others who engage in experimental treatments cause medical professionals great concern as they increase their exposure to unwanted diseases and face needless complications. Evaluating patients by observing their psychological behavior measures well, as it brings humanness to the forefront, as opposed to using predetermined benchmarks that make no distinction based on patients' individual needs.

With chronic kidney disease growing in incidence and with the existing disparity in the ratio of physicians to patients, there is growing concern for physicians, as well as the community, that not each patient is getting enough attention. Physicians in nephrology are looking at ways to address this limitation by developing new sustainable models of health care, conducting training programs for graduates, and increasing awareness of the disease by offering public programs such as early detection to reduce burden of the disease.

Reviewing patients and their method of disease management has shown that many people have been successful in surviving the disease against all odds, and they may be rightly considered as fortunate. Unaware of the consequences of being negligent, many people make huge mistakes and land in situations that reduce their chances of recovery, which is unfortunate. At a time when understanding and sympathy would help in a patient's healing, sometimes family and friends become critical, making the person feel guilty—and slowly the patient withdraws from social life. Over time patients choose to remain isolated, which only allows fear of the disease to develop among the public and the truth to remain shrouded. Physicians are continuously reviewing and formulating changes in their approaches to patient care, minimizing the alarming number of patients who reach critical condition.

The complexity of chronic kidney disease is vastly underestimated in all parts of the world. Our attempt with *Who Lives, Who Dies with Kidney Disease* is to share stories of people who experienced the disease and challenged it. Some of these people lost the battle, while some of them have made history. Through these individual stories, readers will realize the deeper issues related to kidney disease that place patients on tenterhooks. For families of patients, there is an opportunity to discover new things they need to understand about the psychological issues facing their kin. For the very first time, readers will walk along the dark paths that health might take, revealing some huge challenges that could even arrive at their own door if early signs are ignored. As for the medical fraternity, this is another reminder to appropriately raise the alarm for the benefit of communities.

Who Lives, Who Dies with Kidney Disease will initially engage the reader with heartwarming stories. In subsequent chapters, critical information about kidney disease is provided, making this volume a good learning experience. For some it could be the first time encountering basic knowledge and information about the organ and its functioning. Some stories put speculation to rest by focusing on lifestyle changes that help in better health management. Some interesting guidance from patients comes through these stories, and we have provided some first-level tips that could change the mind-sets of patients and families.

In 2006, I met Vasundhara Raghavan when her son Aditya Raghavan was under my care. After a kidney donation in 1999, she developed a deep understanding of the disease and showed considerable interest in kidney-related research studies. This led to our conversations about raising awareness of chronic kidney disease. Interesting developments led to two books being published, with our belief and conviction that the disease needs to be seen from the patient's perspective. Vasundhara actively advocates for awareness of chronic kidney disease management, including dietary issues, in Facebook support groups, and she does considerable work in India.

Who Lives, Who Dies with Kidney Disease and our earlier publication, *Shades of Life: Sublime Joy Is in Living*, attempt to show that a patient may enjoy life beyond dialysis and transplant. The reality is that diet, exercise, and medications play a huge role in disease management. Life is filled with anguish, uncertainty, and intense suffering for patients and their families. Life and existence may have different connotations for different people, but for people dealing with kidney disease, the way they see life is vastly different. Comfort comes through the community's appreciation of the disease, the understanding of the patient's pain, and the community's providing of support as patients face chronic kidney failure with courage.

For the purpose of honoring patient confidentiality and respecting the sensitivities of a few contributors, readers will notice that individual identities are safeguarded. With the consent of those specially interviewed for *Who Lives, Who Dies with Kidney Disease*, their names and photographs are published. All the stories resonate with the trials and tribulations of people from different walks of life. But cost implications of treatments for chronic kidney disease will stand as the single significant differentiator. I am sure that in the future, meeting a person with a chronic kidney condition will touch an emotional chord.

Mohammad Akmal, MD
Professor of Medicine, Keck School of Medicine
University of Southern California

Kidney Lives

Today more than seven billion human beings occupy earth, and this figure grows each minute. Human lives have a definitive purpose. We are to live as characters molded by environmental influences powered by an intuitive mind. Each soul is captive to an exclusively charted path that could cross paths with others on its journey.

Is a pure and perfect life just the figment of an imaginative mind? Or has such a mystical existence been witnessed before and has since undergone a change?

Legend has it that the first humans existed several hundreds of thousands of centuries ago. They walked through green lands, enjoyed the clear blue sky above, and tasted nectar in the sparkling water that gurgled down as a bountiful cascade, meandering over stretches of plains, while solid rock structures symbolized impregnable toughness.

Caught in the fantasy of such a magical past, one wonders when and how imperfection entered the planet's orbit. Gradual conquests by an unworthy character possessing extraordinary manipulative skills and driven by personal ambitions could have spurred the creation of a new domain, where the greed of a silent, purposive intruder systematically planted thoughts, and then acted, to endanger the existence of the innocent breed.

But the air, wind, sun, and water worked as an undercurrent to stretch things further, adding many compulsive distractions mesmerizing to humankind. The world was no longer a realm of fantastical beauty but had become someplace real where human beings exercised their hearts and brains to fathom the turbulence ahead. At each turn, human beings used their superior intellect to overcome and squash this turbulence. But there was much more that awaited them.

Throughout the pages of *Who Lives, Who Dies with Kidney Disease*, we will look at a particular hurdle faced by the human race. Kidney disease is recognized as an ailment that affects people in different ways. How it is contracted, to what extent it affects people, and how well it has been managed over time will be demonstrated. People affected by kidney disease became instruments to overcoming the hurdle placed in this universe at some point of time. These people have given us something special, changes that their passionate ways brought about to life and living.

Early Days

The tide was forever rising and waning. With this, people's lives saw dramatic swings of happiness and despair. For the ones with the ability to smile and take life in their stride, life was enjoyable. They fought challenges; achieved goals by unraveling difficult situations through experimentation; and speculated about the causes of success and failure with equal interest. But some of them belonged to a community that experienced fear, saw adversity, and was confounded by an impenetrable wall that many others managed to conquer with persistence.

What was this invincible power that drove people to madness? One wonders! Nothing was as clear as crystal. Nothing was heard, not even a whimper. Nothing could be understood. All in all, it was mysterious. Pain and uncertainty were crouching in the shadows, waiting to pounce without provocation.

The first time a person confronted kidney disease, was he sworn to silence? Why was it beneath a thick shroud of darkness? Was there anything paranormal about it? Did the earliest incident leave the afflicted person mesmerized? Was it considered to be the devil himself large and daring?

It is said that as early as AD 100, kidney disease was first seen, noticed, and recognized. Stories of events that happened at the Roman baths made the rounds. Some people soaked for long hours and enjoyed being immersed in a great body of water. It was discovered that the cause of kidney disease was a buildup of urea. If one soaked in a bath, the toxicity was removed. This was believed to be as effective as today's dialysis.

Then in AD 1500, the fully recorded case of Stefan Bathory, King of Portland, was later matched with symptoms of polycystic kidney disease. One can safely say that such evidence was recorded because the head of a kingdom showed an unusual health condition. Apart from just being curious, some questioning minds possibly wondered about what had caused the disease.

The history of urinary tract stones began with the history of civilization. In 1901, an English archaeologist named E. Smith detected a bladder stone in a mummy forty-five hundred to five thousand years old in El Amrah, Egypt. Furthermore, treatment for stones was described in ancient Egyptian medical writings from 1500 BC. In 1807, English physician Richard Bright described a disease characterized by edema (swelling of body), the presence of albumin (protein) in the urine, and high blood pressure. This disease was named after him as "Bright's disease."

It isn't an overstatement if one is said to feel marooned when, unceremoniously, a urine-producing organ decides to shut down, either completely stopping urine production or beginning to leak protein into the urine. When this happens, the body enters a totally uncomfortable state of being. Breathlessness, headache, nausea, loss of appetite for food or water, body swelling, and back pain are some promptings that bring to the forefront the uncertainty of life.

The kidneys rank as one the most important organs; they produce urine, eliminate waste products, and synthesize important hormones. Surprisingly, people generally refer to the fullness of their bladder when they have to go to the bathroom and remember the kidney only when they cannot urinate. The Latin term *renes* is related to the English word *reins*, a synonym for "kidneys" in Shakespearean English. The kidneys, always used in the plural (*kelayot*), are mentioned over thirty times in the Bible. In the Pentateuch (the first five books of the Old Testament), the kidneys are cited eleven times in the detailed instructions given for the sacrificial offering of animals at the altar.

The kidney is an organ present in many animals, and in humans the kidneys are located behind the abdominal cavity near the middle of the back below the rib cage. The majority of people possess two kidneys, one on each side, while in rare cases some people have to live with one kidney (either having been born with one or having lost one, either surgically or in an accident). Occasionally, people are born with one or two small and poorly functioning kidneys.

These bean-shaped organs may each be as small as a fist. They possess a million functioning units called nephrons, which are the key performers in the kidney's function.

In humans the kidneys perform a very important function but are sometimes stricken by diverse conditions and disorders. These medical conditions may be congenital or acquired. Some disorders that could cause chronic damage to this organ are diabetes, hypertension, chronic glomerulonephritis (inflammation of the small blood vessels of the kidney), chronic tubulointerstitial nephritis (damage to the tubules and tissues that surround the kidneys called interstitial tissue), polycystic kidney disease, and systemic lupus erythematosus, among many others.

For people affected by chronic kidney disease (CKD), annual treatment of CKD runs into the billions. In some economically advanced countries, patients have the opportunity to decide between hemodialysis and peritoneal dialysis. Furthermore, some eligible patients receive kidney transplantation. In the United States, most kidney transplantations are cadaveric, needing a few years of wait time. Less frequently, some lucky individuals receive a kidney from a relative, and others occasionally get one from an unrelated donor. All these treatment modalities are expensive, are not readily available in most developing countries, and are rationed in the countries with emerging economies.

How likely will it be that a person will recognize the onset of the disease and act quickly? It is widely known that reaction to the disease is generally slow, and the body's slowing down comes many a time with an element of surprise, bordering on a state of shock.

How much related to CKD has changed in the second decade of the twenty-first century?

Kidney failure is widely acknowledged as serious, but today it is the ninth leading death-causing disease. Though the course of the disease has traveled quickly, with treatment breaking many barriers and conquering turbulent waters, there is a growing quest for squashing the finer microscopic elements that keep CKD in the realm of a life-threatening disease. The balance can tip between life and death with even a miniscule dietary change.

We have come a long way since early reporting. Transplants have improved, and dialysis treatments are customized, raising the level of comfort and convenience, allowing for a good lifestyle. Developmental work has improved dialysis machines to make them more efficient in dealing with toxicity, and medications are constantly improved to minimize side effects. However, treatments continue to be cumbersome and expensive. Care providers have found new ways to spread information so that early detection is possible. Many organizations are focused on conducting preventive camps.

The patient, however, continues to remain deeply involved in finding ways to survive. None of the work done by the medical fraternity has much significance. Chronic kidney disease has treatments, but there is no cure.

Mohammad Akmal, MD
Professor Emeritus
Keck School of Medicine
University of Southern California
Los Angeles

PART I: PERSONAL STORIES FROM THE US AND OTHER COUNTRIES

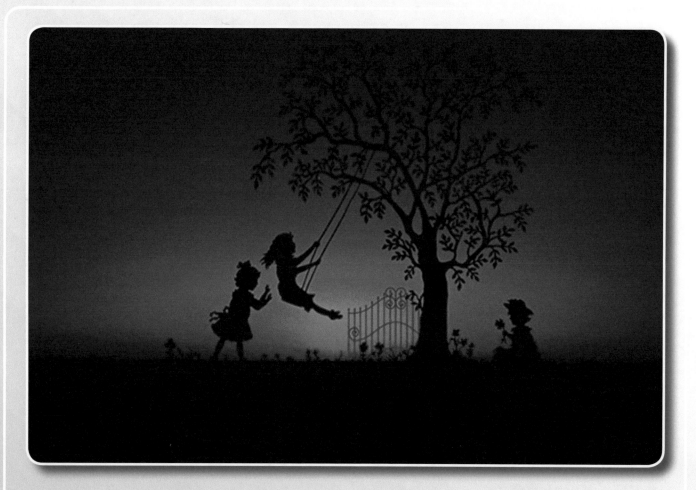

RACING TO WIN – MALU NARA, INDIA

"Malu, I am sure to win. Watch me. Every minute I reach closer to the sky. Here I go!"

With every ounce of energy, I pushed hard on the gravel. My legs were longer than hers; I was plump, more energetic, and more confident. She was my age, smaller and fragile. At that point it didn't bother me that I was flaunting my superior physique and taking full advantage of it.

It was a warm summer day. The air was filled with happiness as school was closed and vacations had just begun. To set the mood and make the whole picture perfect, the birds chirped endlessly, as if a huge forum of speakers were involved in a cheerful debate. I simply loved the garden and the green trees hanging low, swaying with the breeze, in the process losing some precious flaming-red gulmohar flowers.

In my heart, I knew that Malu, for some mysterious reason, was in awe of me. Her noncommunicative ways and soft manner clashed with my overpowering manner, but her docile ways somehow suited me. Who likes to handle a tyrant?

Now that I had made up my mind to win, I busied myself, focusing on pumping my energy to reach my target.

Every time I kicked the mud and moved up, I could see the blue skies and a bird flying by. It was a happy thought sitting on the rough, hard wood and dreaming of winning, while Malu sat tight on her swing in a red and white polka-dotted dress, making little effort to ride high. I could feel my knee-length summery pink and blue floral dress floating merrily as if in celebration.

While I enjoyed myself, laughing mirthfully at her side, there was no sound except the creaky noise of the swing pleading to be lubricated.

Even as I was busy and fully engrossed in play, I saw a manservant rushing toward us, with beads of sweat on his forehead.

"Come. Come. Master is calling you. Some bad news …"

He was breathless. With some agitation he pulled the swings clumsily, using full force to bring them to a rude halt. Malu seemed very eager to leave her perch, but she walked at a slow pace, without even bothering to look back at me.

Unsympathetic, I thought, *What an end to this game! I am surely the winner!* But surprisingly I never gathered up the courage to make a rude comment to her.

Boredom set in as I strolled back to the house, kicking mud as if still in play and angry about having been forced to head back to the house.

Malu's house was a huge mansion standing proud and majestic, occupying a very large green wooded area. It had a red roof, with two robust chimneys emitting smoke whenever the house was filled with guests. Today there was a thin line of smoke making its way to the sky. As it was nearly lunchtime, I wondered if anything exciting would be served for lunch.

Looking up again, I inspected the house closely with admiration. I hoped that my dad would buy such a home with a sprawling garden. I would ask Dad to make a small playhouse on the edge where I could sit for hours, painting or playing Monopoly with my friends. I could even read a book with a cushion tucked under my arm. A mini ladder stacked with some snacks and drinks would make it a complete summer retreat.

Taking a deep breath, I realized this would remain a pipe dream, with no chance of ever becoming real.

As I drew closer, it looked as if the winds had swept the place clean. The veranda looked empty and forlorn. Entering the patio, I had the chilling feeling of being left alone. An enormous silence enshrouded the house. My palms, wet and sticky, closed in a clasp as I stood there for a moment feeling the loneliness of the silence.

I entered and saw the front drawing room had a fan furiously swirling away. I saw that the women were quiet. Their faces looked lost and indifferent, as if they were stranded on an empty road that led nowhere. Suddenly they busied themselves doing trivial things. The stillness was scary, as if time was held back, even though the huge grandfather clock clicked away loudly.

In normal times this room was the busy coffee room. One associated it with strong aromas of freshly brewed coffee and an array of freshly prepared snacks. Some days, the garden tables were laid with a picnic basket, from where Aunt Laxmi and Mom would dig out boxes of exciting food. Oh, what fun those times were!

But now I noticed that everything was starkly different. I saw the room ripped of all happiness, pared down to look drab and insignificant.

Mom pulled me roughly by my forearm and whispered between tight lips, "There's some bad news. Sunder died in the cinema house a few minutes back."

Then looking straight into my eyes, with her index finger held tight against her lips, she said, "Hush."

I looked into her eyes, which were suddenly large with fear and anguish. I was quiet, not daring to do or say anything.

Magically the sun took shelter behind the thick clouds. Darkness cast over the summery house with its teak doors thrown open. The high ventilated ceilings under normal circumstances made the rooms airy and comfortable, but now even the air was heavily doused into silence.

Everyone looked sullen, with no trace of warmth.

This tense atmosphere drew the worst out of me. I felt claustrophobic. On tiptoe, I walked to the window to take refuge behind the heavy curtains. At least the happiness of the world outside could cheer me.

In the garden the swing was slowing down. I knew that soon it would come to a complete halt. Suddenly a car lunged forward out of the driveway and picked up speed. Dad and Malu's father were seated in the rear seat, while the seat beside the driver was occupied by an unfamiliar person.

Their faces each wore a mask of solemnity.

As if perfectly timed, as soon as the car zoomed out of sight, Aunt Laxmi shouted out, tears streaming down her cheeks. Mom did all within her means to pacify her. Aunt ranted, "My poor child ... he was just eighteen years old."

Mom agreed with her and added words to a similar effect.

"What harm did he bring about? Why was he punished?"

Everyone tried hard to console and soothe Aunt Laxmi, but she was inconsolable. My sisters were swarming around Aunt Laxmi, their faces filled with emotion, while Malu stood watching, her eyes wide in surprise and terror.

Late that night as I stirred in bed, I heard Dad whisper to Mom, "Sunder was in the theater watching Alfred Hitchcock's suspense thriller *Psycho*. Doctors think he might have died of shock. It is a horror film. Suddenly a chair swings and there's a skeleton, you know."

He grunted and chuckled loud, while Mom chuckled softly.

He continued with his suppressed whisper: "These young people! Why should they go to adult movies?"

Then after a few minutes, letting out a deep breath, he said "Why would he want to see such scary movies?"

The truth was out in a few days.

Sunder had been declared dead after his kidneys had completely shut down.

With his untimely death, a few things happened. Our visits to Uncle Nara's became occasional and slowly tapered off to naught. The family in mourning found it hard to come to terms with their first child's abrupt exit from the world. They needed time and space to heal.

The fun times of family picnics were now just some vague memories of the past.

Dad would bring fresh news now and then.

It was almost an annual event. Five of six kids in that family were sucked in by renal failure. It was a mystery. We were clueless about what had caused the disease that dwelled in the bodies of individuals we met almost every weekend. Among the kids who disappeared in that household was my dear friend Malu. All memories of our playtimes were sealed in a protective cage in my brain's gray cells.

In those years, Uncle Nara slowly dug his own grave. He was an ace marketing manager in the petroleum industry who seemed too shocked by his inability to use his resources to change the destiny of even one of his dying children. Aunt Laxmi protectively held her last surviving child close to her bosom as if challenging the demons, as any mother would, guarding him from a powerful destructive opponent.

In the dimmed lighting of our household, everyone spoke of these tragedies in undertones lined with deep fear. All I knew was that with kidney failure, people just died. I had to grow up before I could learn more.

This happened in 1962 in Mumbai, India's premier city, where doctors had only some basic information on renal failure. But there were lots of reservations about discussing the matter. Treatment was explained in as vague a manner as possible, with the doctors exhibiting anxiety and showing a lack of understanding of how to handle the patients. They had a limited scope when it came to providing any positive solution. Limited knowledge and limited resources! Much has happened since then to the renal world thanks to science, through clinical work, coupled with people's greater understanding of the disease.

Nephrology, the study of renal disease, became popular in First World countries such as the United States and the United Kingdom in the 1960s. With a ripple effect, organizations were formed to do further research, provide support, and make treatments for this life-threatening disease available. Not much has changed worldwide when it comes to this disease, as far as the fear factor goes. Life seems unpredictable. Despite uncertainty hanging in the air, researchers have found many solutions for people who have kidney disease to live good-quality lives.

Vasundhara Raghavan

"CAN I BE OF ANY HELP, BROTHER?" – R. AND H.

When World War II ended, a silence settled over the world, giving people an opportunity to resume their lives. Families whose members were victims of the war had to shed the memories of their loved ones and build their lives on the hope of a better future. They understood that time would heal their wounds. While parts of the world busied itself with the serious business of developing a country or focusing on personal growth, some unsettled matters bubbled in a hot pot.

One such lingering problem rocked Korea. Ruled by Japan from 1910 until the end of World War II in 1945, Korea finally surrendered to US administrators, who then divided the Korean Peninsula along the 38th parallel. This division meant that the Republic of Korea was supported by the United States with allied nations under the aegis of the United Nations, and the Democratic People's Republic of Korea was led by the People's Republic of China, with military and material aid from the USSR.

Then the constant tussle between the two powers, the United States and the Union of Soviet Socialist Republics, each with a different ideology, tore apart the fabric of Korea. North Korea had a single planned development, whereas South Korea followed a democratic government and a free market economy. Living conditions were not normal and were subjected to lots of pressure from the superpowers.

The bubble burst on June 25, 1950, when the Korean War broke out between North and South Korea. The US military called able-bodied men to serve in the war at various military posts.

Among these servicemen were twin brothers H. and R. One had received a posting in the coast guard, and the other had been selected by the army and was sent out to Germany. The brothers had left their father, their brother V., and a younger sister, S., to join the services.

It was fortunate for H. and R. that they were far away from the intense war activity. They had escaped the travails of living in a high-pressure war zone; they were not consumed by a thirst for human blood; their sleep at night was peaceful and not interrupted by the hissing sounds of bullets screeching by; they were not terrorized by the oppression or starvation normally dealt to prisoners of war; and they were not subject to unscrupulous massacre. Their time in the service was very easy compared to that of many who were deeply involved in the war.

The war ended in July 1953.

The brothers planned their return home with their humanity intact, holding love in their hearts. During the war their father had died. Because they were motherless, the family would now live with an aunt and an uncle.

On the scheduled date, H. had arrived. The siblings and caregivers were concerned that R. had not yet arrived.

Instead, a shocking letter arrived from Marine Hospital, Chicago, stating that they had detained R., who was diagnosed with chronic kidney disease and was facing disorientation. The family was alarmed. How could a normal, healthy young man suddenly be so disoriented? The letter mentioned that toxins had accumulated in R.'s blood, manifesting in psychotic behavior.

Suddenly, R.'s health and his survival posed a far greater uncertainty than had the days he'd spent serving in the war. R.'s death seemed to the family most imminent and a logical conclusion.

Suddenly the tides changed. Concerned about R.'s condition, V., as the eldest sibling, spoke to the doctor at the US Public Health Service about what could be done to save R. The doctor recalled pioneering work being done in Peter Bent Brigham Hospital, Boston, Massachusetts, where the first transplant had been done in 1950 on a forty-four-year-old. Unfortunately the organ was rejected. (Immunosuppressant therapy was nonexistent at that time.)

The doctor explained at length that in case of a tissue mismatch, the body considers the transplanted organ to be a foreign object and rejects it. It dawned on the doctor that organ donation between twins would not be subject to tissue compatibility issues. This triggered a new thought. H. elected to donate.

When they were admitted to the hospital for the transplant, H. spent time recalling all that had been discussed and how things had panned out in those early months. *I want R. back, safe and in normal health. But is this experimental surgery worth it?*

Meetings with the doctors, along with serious discussions involving his life and future, had tired him. *Let me get it done and be in peace.*

H. leaned back and closed his eyes. His first thought was to save R. He was keen and excited. But also he was very confused. H. felt a knot in the pit of his stomach. The thought that he was healthy and that they would cut him open and take out one of his organs was alarming. Deep down he felt some fear. The only surgery H. had ever had was an appendectomy, which he had not liked very much.

To H., a kidney transplant was more in the realm of science fiction. He'd never dreamed he would be a participant in such a tale. All throughout he had been in a dilemma; his mind had engaged itself in conflicting thoughts. He wanted to help his brother, but how would he go through such a major surgery?

Suddenly he was disturbed by a faint knock that he chose to ignore. Shifting to a more comfortable position, he focused on his thoughts.

During family discussions, some worrying aspects had come to the forefront. Clearly by now, the anxiety was for both the donor and the recipient. Appropriately, the family had raised pertinent questions, which the doctors had fielded.

"What is the life expectancy of a person with one kidney?"

It was not difficult for the doctor to give a pat response, but it occurred to him that getting a third party's assurance would break down the reservations.

The doctor approached insurance companies for access to actuarial tables. After lengthy study, the insurance companies made an unusual discovery and reported that there was no increased risk of death when living with one kidney. They talked of people born with a single kidney, which had an incidence of one in one thousand people.

The knock on the door grew more insistent. H.'s brow creased in slight irritation. *This reflection is helping me clear my head … It is the last few hours before dawn, and then …*

Breathing deeply, he responded in a clear, loud voice: "Please come in. The door is open."

The night nurse entered the dark room and switched on the light. With a bright smile, she broke the heavy silence by announcing, "Checkup time!"

Noisily placing her nursing tray on the bedside table, she popped the thermometer into H.'s mouth, pulling out a note that she then placed within his easy reach.

As she finished checking his vital signs, she cleared her throat noisily. Looking straight into his eyes, she said, "Your brother sent it to you."

Reaching out, H. picked up the note and read it slowly, once, twice: "Get out of here and go home."

He crushed the note in his right palm, his tight fist revealing pale white knuckles. He was unhappy that his brother was still wavering, in spite of repeated assurances and after the topic had been endlessly discussed and was concluded and sealed.

The nurse stood watching him, waiting for the next reaction. Scared and worried about having been the bearer of a letter sensitive to timing, she was wary. *Did the contents disturb the young man? Oh why, why, did I take this risk? The doc will be furious!*

She stood silently wringing her hands, all the time praying. The surgery was scheduled for early the next morning. Hopefully she had not crushed the opportunity. So many people waited eagerly for this surgery.

Now have I endangered it?

Over the past few days, she had watched the brothers battle out their emotions. She continued to chew her lower lip, as was her habit when facing uncomfortable moments.

Sitting upright in his bed, H. collected his thoughts.

Picking up a notepad, he began scribbling. Thoughts of his brother lying on the hard uncomfortable bed, with pain keeping him restless, suddenly made his expression soften. In that moment of calm, his mind received some clarity. With a lot more enthusiasm, he wrote his brother a message, one that he would be proud of for a long time to come: "I am here and I am going to stay."

Folding the crisp note, H. handed it to the nurse, saying, "Madam, please give this note to my brother immediately, before he retires."

The night was young but strung high with emotion. One brother's mind swayed, suggesting no surgery, and the other emphatically knocked down the former's decision. In a glorious moment, calm was established. Their worlds were put to rest as soon as the decision was cemented.

For a long time after the nurse left, H. sat thinking. He remembered the prelude to this moment, including his family's involvement in the decision.

At one point, another thought had crossed the mind of one of his family members. Without much ado, the query was placed before the doctors: "What are the chances of subsequent disease affecting the remaining kidney?"

Recognizing the family's mental turmoil, one of the doctors had explained, "Most common types of renal disease affect both kidneys simultaneously. The most critical conditions affecting a solitary kidney are cancer and trauma, both of which fortunately are rare."

These explanations had brought great relief to the troubled family, who were looking for foolproof solutions. Now with full confidence, they were excited to go ahead and do the surgery.

The matter rested thereafter with the doctors.

A huge responsibility had been placed on the doctors to plan and execute the surgery with precision.

Before attempting to open a healthy young man, the doctors wanted to do two things:

- complete a trial run
- graft a skin transplant from recipient to donor

As plans were afoot, for the first time the doctors were stumped by an unusual situation, requiring them to revisit their role.

Loyalties were now divided. There would be two people on the surgery table—one who needed the operation to save his life, and one who had agreed to help.

Whom would the doctors go to bat for first?

The obvious thing to do was to put all their energies toward the cure of the patient who suffered from physical pain and traumatic episodes. After all, weren't the doctors aware of R.'s deteriorating condition, knowing that any delay could cause the loss of a precious life?

Most tempting to them was the aspect of testing out their theory of similar twins having a 100 percent tissue match, which could be a reason for long survival rates for patients who have had a kidney transplant!

The doctors agreed about their primary duty toward the patient.

But while calculating the nitty-gritty of the surgeries, their minds had opened up and they deliberated on their role of protecting the healthy man to whom the extensive surgical procedure would bring no real benefit. They found it unfortunate that his life was about to be endangered to the extent that any surgery endangers life.

Troubled faces around the room suddenly showed a qualitative shift in the doctors' thinking. Surprisingly, they had unilaterally agreed that the healthy person was the one whose life should be watched out for.

Only after several series of consultations within the hospital and several done externally, including with legal counsel, had the doctors made their decision. Yes, they would do the surgery with methodical planning, minute detailing, and complete validation of results.

Though the surgery would be establishing a new procedure that would change the world's perception of kidney disease and bring the doctors personal repute, the prospect for them dimmed when they considered the consequences of putting a healthy life in danger.

Suddenly all this reflection was tiring to H. He looked at his watch and realized it was close to midnight. He should rest and be ready early for the surgery. He got up, stretched his body, and flexed his muscles. Now he felt relaxed. His brother's last message asking him to go home hadn't deterred him from doing what he had set out to do.

Feeling calmer, he settled down for a restful sleep. In the morning there would be so much activity and excitement. The air was heavy with an element of suspense and curiosity. How successful would this experimental surgery be?

The doctors knew this wasn't an experiment, but a natural transition to the development of best medical practices, taking surgery to its next level, from partial to confirmed success. A transplant without immunosuppressant drugs needed a 100 percent tissue match, so the twin brothers' case became a critical clinical study.

Even as the brother was being readied to donate his kidney, intensive study to get the procedure right was taking place at the lead surgeon's office. The doctor looked at the minute details. Small mistakes could mean the balance could tip the other way. The doctor made copious notes for a clinical report that would serve as the blueprint for the surgical procedure. Risky surgery needed meticulous planning.

Ingenious thinking was another highlight of the doctor's experimental surgery. To establish veracity of his theory that there was 100 percent match between the twins' tissues, the doctor, as an additional safeguard, arranged to have both donor and recipient fingerprinted at the local police station.

A newspaper reporter saw hospital staff making secret visits to the police station. Everything was being done in a hush. This raised a suspicion in the newspaper office. Suddenly it caused a stir.

What is the strange business happening between the police station and hospital? was the question in many minds.

News leaked out of "unusual happenings" at the Brigham Hospital.

Slowly the story came out. News of the transplant became a sensation.

There was a broadcast on a radio station. People tuned in to get every bit of information they could about the transplant. It became a daily broadcast until the transplant was completed. This added pressure to the surgical team to perform successfully.

As to the ethical part, the surgeons maintained a high level of transparency in all discussions with the donor. In spite of its being their first possible chance for a successful transplant, the team placed all facts before the donor and his family, leaving them to make the decision without any remorse. These factors built confidence in the donor and the public.

It is commendable that a detailed and systematic approach document was prepared introducing the clinical technique for a successful organ transplant. Minute details of the surgery were recorded, telling us the time taken for each step of the process, for example, the donor's kidney, wrapped in a wet, cold towel, was transported in a sterile basin. This establishes the fact that the surgeon had highly creative thinking, which when combined with proactive measures made this a winning discovery.

With such meticulous planning, at the end of the day a template for future transplants was ready.

Procedure: Identical-twin kidney transplant

Date: December 23, 1954

Institution: Peter Bent Brigham Hospital, Boston, Massachusetts

The doctor masterminded a transplant that made history: the first long-surviving kidney transplant patient without immunosuppressant medications. The fact that the tissue of monozygotic (identical) twins was compatible was used to increase our understanding of how much relief this type of surgery can bring.

The story is extraordinary on many levels, as follows:

- H. offered his kidney when there were no known success rates for long-term successful organ donations. His offer was self-motivated and purely an act of love.
- R. survived the transplant and lived for eight years thereafter.

- The men's parents were not alive to see this great feat performed by the operating surgeon, or the love and bond between their adult children.
- It became a winning experiment, making history in the field of nephrology. It was "this magical first transplant" that paved the way for organ transplants in other parts of the world. Kidney patients saw an opportunity for relief and to lead normal lives!

H. was driven by a sense of duty. Without batting an eyelid, he agreed to donate his kidney. The procedure was, in his words, "in the realm of science fiction." The doctor was honored with a Nobel Prize for Medicine in 1990.

Source: Dr. Joseph Murray, *Surgery of the Soul: Reflections on a Curious Career* (Sagamore Beach, MA: Science History Publications, 2001).

The story has been dramatized to showcase this spectacular case.

EARLY LESSONS – SUSAN AND RICHARD

She stood near the toilet and saw that her urine had small spots of blood in it. Eyes wide with wonder, she inspected the toilet seat. It had no trace of blood. But she was confused. What was this? Twisting her frock at the hem, she stepped out of the bathroom nervously. But her anxiety was momentary. No sooner than she heard her brother shout out to her, she tossed her head, and her fear went away. "Susan, come soon," he'd said. "It's now your turn."

Susan ran back, excited. She wanted to catch the thief soon in the game they were playing. The last time her chance had been squashed. What a shame!

The next day, when she peeked into the toilet bowl, it was the same thing. Her urine had small specks of blood in it. Now her fear resurfaced.

She walked out quietly and went straight to her mother.

"Mother … Mother …" She stopped, not clear about what to say next.

"What is it, Susan? Be quick. I'm busy. I need to finish this fast and get ready for dinner." Susan's mother was busy wrapping up her unfinished desk work. Seeing Susan silent, hesitant, and looking a bit confused, her mother got anxious.

Fortunately Susan was extremely smart. Realizing it was best to show evidence, she took her mother's hand and walked her to the toilet.

What her mother saw drew the breath out of her. Settling six-year-old Susan on a high stool, she asked some questions. Susan could answer all but one: What had happened to her?

The next day they took the road to the nearest clinic. After several days of physical examinations and unique tests being performed, one doctor detected something far more serious than Susan could comprehend, let alone handle. What the doctor said was a shocking revelation even for the parents.

"I think Susan has some kind of kidney disease. It is known as Bright's disease or glomerulonephritis. At some point her kidneys may shut down completely. Until then we need to take extreme care. Hopefully it will happen progressively."

Susan's mom realized the enormity of the challenge that lay ahead.

This will be huge, very huge. How will I save my daughter from this insurmountable disease?

This happened during a time when little was known of the disease. But with some guidance from the physician, Susan's mother established basic precautions for living with the disease.

This early introduction of safe measures proved useful, as Susan managed to hold her life together for nearly four decades. Was it a streak of courage that held her life together? Was she prepared for what was just around the bend and knew the next great agent of change in her life? Was it pure luck? It is anyone's guess. Everything is mere speculation.

Susan married George, an engineer, who, being highly educated, had a better understanding of the seriousness of the disease. This union possibly made a great impact on how Susan's disease was managed.

George and Susan were overjoyed with the birth of their son Frank and his younger brother, Richard, in 1952 and 1956, respectively. Even as their lives filled with joy, tides of pain lashed the walls of their strong fortress, threatening to shatter it.

At an early age, traces of blood were found in Richard's urine. Susan picked up the cue and knew where this was heading. Understanding basic issues, being able to manage situations, and wearing brave smiles, the couple encouraged Richard and educated him on what to expect.

In a few years Susan developed high blood pressure, which culminated in nephrosclerosis (hardening of the nephrons), as revealed by a kidney biopsy.

In 1983, at twenty-seven years of age, Richard had an episode of gout that showed him the dark face of his kidney disease. Doctors confirmed it was glomerulonephritis.

The next eight years saw a slow but steady decline in Richard's kidney function. As if cocooned in a world of his own, he slogged on to graduate with a doctorate in philosophy. He became an assistant professor. His family had an addition at this stage, as his wife gave him a baby. Richard's life seemed blissful. In the darkness of a closet, between piles of linen, the disease lay trapped. Richard let it lie there while he remained on a low-protein, low-salt diet, which helped delay kidney failure by a few years. But the disease sneered at him, kept him constantly tired, and was slowly growing to overwhelm him.

In 1986 Susan's kidney showed signs of shutting down. She started dialysis a year later.

It seemed the mother–son duo went through the stages of disease with one leading and the other following at arm's length. There was a show of courage and forbearance, masking deep emotional turbulence that lay below the surface.

The year 1990 saw both mother and son at the dialysis center.

Figure 1. Mother and son's matching dates for disease, dialysis, and transplant

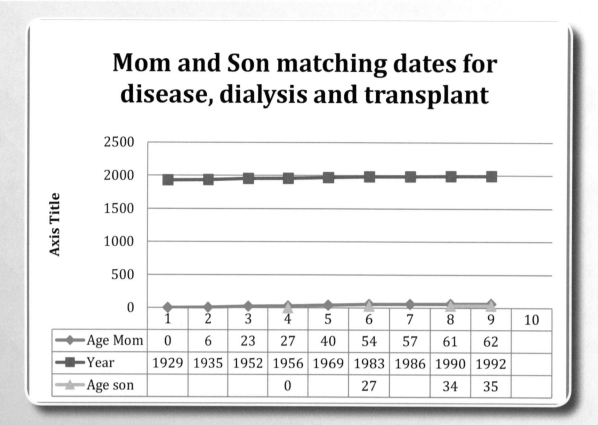

Mom and Son matching dates for disease, dialysis and transplant

	1	2	3	4	5	6	7	8	9	10
◆ Age Mom	0	6	23	27	40	54	57	61	62	
■ Year	1929	1935	1952	1956	1969	1983	1986	1990	1992	
▲ Age son				0		27		34	35	

Susan was born in 1929. In 1935, her kidney disease was detected. In 1952 she gave birth to her first son, and her second son, Richard, was born in 1956. She suffered from high blood pressure in 1964 high BP. In 1986, it was confirmed that her kidneys were shutting down. She underwent dialysis from 1987 to 1992 dialysis. In 1992 she received a kidney transplant.

Richard was born in 1956. In 1983, it was confirmed that he had kidney disease. He began dialysis in 1990, and in 1992 he received a kidney transplant.

George had a formidable task, namely, saving lives of two very dear people, his wife and son—one who had seen different facets of the life-threatening disease, and the other who carried hope in his young, eager eyes. This meant that George had to be mentally alert enough to maintain stability and find the latest medical advancements.

Susan's foray into dialysis began with continuous ambulatory peritoneal dialysis (CAPD), which she underwent in order to live a better lifestyle. But she experienced seven episodes of peritonitis. Under duress she was compelled to change to hemodialysis, which meant greater dietary restrictions and a greatly diminished lifestyle. Her diet was strict, and she had to keep her fluid intake low. She was on high doses of erythropoietin (EPO), yet she remained tired, fought sleeplessness, and developed a cough and breathing problems caused by fluid buildup. High blood pressure was a major stumbling block where listing for organ transplant was concerned. Many prominent medical centers evaluated her and subsequently rejected her candidacy.

George had to find that one missing link that would nail down the solution to their problems and bring long-lasting relief for the whole family.

George's unequivocal support through Susan's toughest periods can only be imagined. Likely that he watched her in pain, helped her to lift CAPD bags, or looked out for when the cycler machine beeped. One can guess that there were both sad and happy periods and imagine that his waking hours were singularly directed toward securing the lives of two family members facing grave health conditions.

In Susan's eyes, pain would be visible, and as a parent her disappointment quite expected seeing her son stretched out on a bed in the clinic, being dialyzed with needles pricking him. No matter that Richard may have consoled her on many occasions. But she knew well what those tubes did in the process of bringing out blood to clean it, while the person was strapped down. She knew well the nauseous feeling, the cramps, and the feeling of lowness.

The person who bore it silently while watching from the distance and mulling it all over was Richard's elder brother, Frank. As a son and brother, all throughout his growing years he had witnessed how the disease had troubled his mother. And in later years, his kid brother, Richard, joined her brigade. How it impacted Frank's life was never a subject of discussion. But it is true that every family member is deeply affected by the strain of the disease.

In a unique manner, Frank chose to play monitor, keeping tabs on the disease's progression. At an appropriate moment, he encouraged Susan to undergo an evaluation for transplant. But her uncontrolled blood pressure became an impediment and the centers discouraged her, explaining that such surgery could prove disastrous for her.

Richard managed his disease responsibly, bringing some sense of relief to his parents.

If one peeked through their window, one would notice a busy household. But if one were intent, it would not escape their notice that most of the activity in the household surrounded the patients and their medical treatments. Stepping back, the observer would heave a deep breath and marvel at the family's determination to learn new ways to understand and accept their life's challenges.

Frank was considered to be a probable donor for Richard, but initial tests showed that the brothers' blood types did not match. Providence had it that George's kidney matched with Richard's. And then, with some persuasion, the center agreed to allow Frank to donate a kidney to Susan, as they had the same blood type. Miraculously the doctors were willing to go ahead with Susan's transplant!

On July 30, 1992, Richard had his transplant. His mother had hers two months later.

The fear that her age would cause her body to reject the transplanted kidney drove Susan (sixty-two years of age) and George (sixty-four years of age) to work toward getting physically fit. They paved the way for changing opportunities into destinies.

As he looks back, Richard appreciates the kind of change the disease made to his life. The pain and suffering, being part and parcel of the disease, groomed him to be a far greater human being with compassion for and understanding of human lives. He truly values the gift of the disease.

Factors that contributed to this family's achievement are as follows:

- opening doors to knowledge
- being aware of the issues related to kidney failure
- forming emotional bonds and appreciating the intensity of pain the two family members were in
- embarking on the road to kidney transplant single-mindedly
- having no compulsions and no differing views
- being clear on the single purpose of life
- having a dedicated commitment among family members

After the transplant, the family shared their experiences with transplants and explained how the surgeries had enriched their lives. Each member of the family approached the topic from his or her own perspective. Their aim was to encourage living donor transplants.

_____

This story is based on information supplied by George, with whom the author was in touch until 2013. The family had a website that provided updates. Susan's death, unrelated to the kidney disease, was shared at some point. The website has recently been disabled. Out of respect for privacy, names have been changed.

COURAGE GROWS WITH COMPLICATIONS
– KELLY FRANCIS

"Mom, I will be late getting home tonight. It's girls' night out," Kelly said nonchalantly.

It took a moment for her to realize that she was being abrupt and rude. Biting her lower lip, she realized how deeply her attitude would hurt her mother. Wiping clean every trace of indifference from her behavior, she flashed a bright smile as she walked up to her mother. She hugged her mother briefly, and said in an excited voice, "Mom, I forgot to mention it earlier. Eleanor has a wonderful late evening sale to launch their new season collection. It's tomorrow at 7:00 p.m. … Shall we do dinner at the Wok and then shop at the store? I haven't been there in a while."

"Ah, that will be wonderful, Kelly. I've been meaning to do some clothes shopping before going on my holiday."

"So it's a plan, Mom. Let's do it. I will ask Myra to book a table at 6:00 p.m."

Picking up her car keys, Kelly looked back and added, "I will be back by eleven at the latest. Good night, Mom."

Kelly walked out swiftly. She was late by a few minutes for the blind date. Lisa and Henry would join them later at the pub.

Her mother was glad that she and Kelly had planned a dinner for the next day. After a while, she went back to her evening routine and became thoughtful. Seeing Kelly young, beautiful, and so full of life always made her happy.

But in the past few months she had noticed something. She was unable to understand what had happened. In her quieter moments, she consoled herself that Kelly was no longer a kid, and these changes were part of emerging as a young woman holding a top position in the fashion world.

No matter what, she felt some discomfort that she couldn't disclose to anyone.

At times she blamed Kelly for her great weakness for partying heavily. Weekends were completely spent with friends, with little rest before the start of another long week. Her work as head of sales and marketing at Elitist kept her busy on weekdays. She worked hard for long hours and then returned home late, exhausted.

Kelly loved her work.

What a wonderful work environment! It was chic and modern—the most happening place for young go-getters. People were drawn there by the creative layouts, the exciting offers, and the wonderful selection of fabric textures and accessories. In addition to organizing the store displays and promotions, Kelly's knowledge of designs made her a go-to person for sourcing products to many suppliers.

Kelly was a decision maker, and her skills were amply recognized and rewarded by her employers. Her dedication and involvement made her indispensable. Work was very stressful, but she managed it well.

There was one thing that she regretted, though.

With such a demanding schedule, she was unable to find enough time to spend with her mother. She hated that her being busy with work and extracurricular activities meant at times neglecting her mom, her best friend and mentor. She never forgot how hard her Mom had worked, making many personal sacrifices, to see that Kelly got an education and graduated.

Kelly's personal ambitions and need for a life partner had fueled many of her preoccupations. She dreamed of opening her own store under a joint venture with a famed designer. She was at a high point in her life and wanted to accomplish a lot.

The next morning, with her mind racing, one hand on the car's steering wheel and the other busy getting her phone, Kelly called her mom. "Hey, Mom. So you remember our evening's program?"

"Hey, Kelly. Yes, I'm looking forward to it. I will drive over at a quarter to six."

"See you, Mom!"

It was a hectic workday for Kelly as they had annual stocktaking.

Before midday, surprisingly she was exhausted. Her weakness persisted until noon, at which time it looked like she would collapse. With great difficulty, she picked up her cell phone and dialed the last number she had called.

"Something very funny has happened. Since this morning I have felt very low and exhausted. I am unable to do any work!"

"Kelly, it may be your partying late last night."

She whispered back, "Mom, I am too weak to fight with you … I have no energy left."

"Kelly, I think you need to get yourself checked out. Go to Good Samaritan and see a doctor. I will meet you there."

Taking her cue from her mother's advice, Kelly left work, excusing herself for a few hours. The hospital was just two blocks away. She parked her car with great difficulty and was almost swooning when she entered the lobby. Though extremely tired, she managed to fill out the paperwork with her personal information and insurance details.

Her mother walked in, saying, "There you are! Oh, Kelly, you do look pale."

Just then the assistant called, "Kelly Francis!"

The doctor was friendly and asked many questions. Kelly answered politely, though she wanted to just get some quick fix to her health problem and run back to the store.

The doctor put her through several tests. They met again after a couple of hours. Studying the reports, the doctor seemed disappointed when he said, "I am sorry, but things do not seem good as far as your health is concerned. Your blood pressure is very high. The blood test shows high levels of creatinine. It looks like you are heading toward kidney failure."

"Doctor, what is creatinine? I mean, what does it do?" Kelly asked vaguely, as this word rang no bells for her.

"Ms. Francis, creatinine is a chemical waste product in the blood that goes to the kidneys, which release it in the urine. Levels of creatinine indicate how well the kidneys are functioning. So one may say your kidney function is impaired."

Twenty-year-old Kelly was too stunned to utter a word.

As soon as she collected her thoughts, she asked the one question that was bothering her: "How did it happen? What triggered it?"

The doctor nodded. "You need to undergo more tests. Get a sonography and a chest x-ray. Then we will have a clear picture."

The initial tests were enough to create panic in mother and daughter. Kelly was distraught and had no idea how to manage her health. Gathering all her courage to find solutions, Kelly's mother started discussing with the doctor the kind of treatments that Kelly would need in order to remain well. Even after receiving the results of a battery of tests, the doctor could not draw any conclusion as to what had caused the kidney failure. But it was confirmed that Kelly would be starting dialysis very soon.

With her mother by her side, Kelly took stock of the situation.

She studied the various options for dialysis and decided to go for peritoneal dialysis (PD). With PD she would be able to manage her life and enjoy a reasonable degree of comfort.

Gradually Kelly's life changed. Gone were the days of hectic partying. Her health care occupied most of her time. To begin with, her hemoglobin was low. To treat her anemic condition, she was given erythropoietin (an anemia-correcting hormone) at regular intervals.

But as one problem got resolved, another cropped up. These troubles were like unwelcome guests knocking at her door now and then.

Several weeks after her initial diagnosis, Kelly noticed a change in her skin. It had become so itchy that it grew rough and red. Applying calamine lotion gave her only temporary relief.

Her blood test helped to catch the culprit. Her phosphorus level was rising rapidly. She sought to manage this problem with the help of food charts given to her by her doctor showing which foods were high in phosphorus. These kept her worried, but she found it very difficult to put the good information to use. Finally she approached a dietician and explained her problem.

"From your blood report, it is clear that higher levels of phosphorus are creating the problem. This means you need to restrict intake of foods high in phosphorus. Without limiting foods with high phosphorus content, you'll land yourself in a serious problem. Lowering phosphorus will stop this itchiness. Read these," she said, handing Kelly some leaflets.

Drawing her into the conversation, the dietician asked Kelly to share the details of her diet.

Though Kelly was concerned with her health and the severe itching, when the dietician probed into her eating habits, she grew hesitant. Gradually she let the cat out of the bag. Kelly loved her comfort foods, which included pizza and cola. The dietician suggested the option of low-fat cream cheese as a substitute for cheese, to be eaten on toast with vegetables like lettuce, bell peppers, onions, and cucumbers. She suggested limiting consumption of such fast foods by adopting a healthier diet. She talked of whole grains and fresh vegetables and suggested snacks like carrot sticks, apples, and simple cucumber sandwiches to satisfy hunger and also improve health. She concluded, "A little management of diet through restriction of certain foods such as dairy products will help in curbing the rampantly increasing phosphorus. Additionally, your doctor will prescribe phosphorus binders that will bind the phosphorus in your intestines. This will help you."

Much as she tried, Kelly's phosphorus level remained unrestrained. It was tough for her to choose alternative foods to reduce her phosphorus levels.

Problems escalated for Kelly when new issues developed. Her blood test gave another alert—elevated parathyroid hormone. This spelled a problem, exposing her to associated complications that could end in bone disease, skin problems, anemia, and cardiovascular disease.

She was advised to undergo medical therapy for lowering the level of her parathyroid hormone.

It was midmorning on a summer day. Kelly had just left the doctor's clinic and was feeling cold. She decided to go to the cafeteria for a hot drink and spend time trying to understand where her life was heading. She sat at a corner table in the hospital's cafeteria, huddled up to keep warm, feeling burdened with the pressures of health and life in general. At this hour there was a thin crowd. Sipping her coffee, she let her thoughts go back to a past that she had forsaken long ago when caught by the fangs of chronic kidney disease. *I was always the author of my destiny until that point. Now life is slipping away so fast. So many minor issues turning to major health problems are coming up. Will I ever regain control of my health?*

Tears were threatening to flow as she saw it as a losing game. *This is something beyond my capacity to understand. It is huge! How will I retrace my steps and regain my stability? I had built my life from naught; I was the sole provider for Mom and me. What will happen to us?*

The coffee did little to give her any peace. Collecting her bag, she left the hospital, resigning to let destiny direct and lead her.

Very soon it became obvious that, in spite of her efforts, there was no way Kelly could get a handle on the vagrant blood levels. Slowly she was drawn toward the prospect of major surgeries.

She developed hyperparathyroidism. Tumors developed in her parathyroid glands, an indication that her calcium levels had peaked. To make some sense out of her health, which was taking many plunges, and set her free, it would be necessary to remove three and a half of four of her parathyroid glands. With several weeks of calcium and vitamin D therapy, her condition stabilized and her phosphorus levels showed some improvement.

There is no limit to the pain and suffering of kidney patients. Kelly was put to her next test. Years of peritoneal dialysis wore her peritoneum lining thin. This came to her attention when she started experiencing night sweats, fatigue, abdominal pain, and intermittent fever.

The nephrologist suspected abdominal tuberculosis. He arranged peritoneoscopy (a procedure to look into her abdomen to evaluate the condition of the peritoneal membrane). Under the powerful machine, the membrane looked abnormal. A biopsy of an abdominal gland showed that she had tuberculosis (TB).

Treatment for TB was commenced, but a serious liver complication developed as a result of the TB drug. Kelly was ordered a long hospital stay to make full recovery possible. The nephrologist permitted alternative medication to her TB regimen, to accelerate recovery.

Though she was very comfortable with PD, Kelly's peritoneal membrane was unable to survive this onslaught, so she switched to hemodialysis (HD).

Kelly bravely made it through various complications that rocked her life. She remained cheerful throughout. With eyes filled with hope and dreams, she now awaits a kidney for transplant.

***

For a person affected by kidney disease, diet plays a great role. Limiting foods high in phosphorus might have helped Kelly. Making the right food choices is a science in itself. It takes a great deal of dedicated attention to get it right. In the case of excess phosphorus, which cannot be removed by a diseased kidney, the chance that it will affect the bones and parathyroid glands makes it an important mineral to watch out for so a slow-performing kidney is not burdened. Eating forbidden food, as one may refer to chocolates, cheese, meat, and other foods high in phosphorus, must be seriously curtailed to avoid adverse health conditions.

Judging people who fail to manage their blood levels is easy from the comfort of our armchairs, but achieving the balance in reality is very tough. One has to deal with sodium, phosphorus, potassium, blood sugar, and protein. In specific cases, minerals like magnesium might also be an issue. With a diseased kidney unable to perform its function completely, the balanced load can tip very fast. Health is unpredictable. But it's important to understand that managing a dialysis-friendly diet is a huge challenge for everyone.

Tom Carter stood watching his daughter Susan leave with her baby.

Ha! Now Mary and I can spend a quiet evening together—maybe have a cold beer and some baked pita chips, olives, and salsa. These thoughts raced through his brain as he smacked his dry lips and sank comfortably into his black leather study chair.

I need to complete this assignment quickly, he reminded himself, as he hooked his reading spectacles on the bridge of his nose and opened a document on his Mac.

Suddenly it seemed as if words were just tumbling out from the screen.

"Now I can do without such interruptions! My spectacles need cleaning." Reaching for a tissue, he worked aggressively, irritation evident on his otherwise calm face.

His spectacles were cleaned, but without any improved result.

"What's wrong with me? Why is my vision suddenly blurred?"

With growing fear, he realized that something was seriously wrong with his eyes. Every time he attempted to read, he had a similar experience. Sinking back in his chair, he grappled with trying to recover his balance. But forces unknown to him squashed his feeble, panicked attempts, taking his body into the depths of darkness.

It was well after seven when Mary entered his study.

"Tom! Why in heavens are you working in darkness?"

Normally, he would have let out a loud chuckle at being disturbed or being reprimanded. But he met Mary with silence. She groped for the switch. Finding it, she turned on his table lamp. Under its brilliance, she saw that Tom was slumped, his shoulders hunched.

She rushed across to Tom, anxiously shaking him to bring him out of his stupor. But he was unmoved. Her heart was in a state of flutter as she dialed 911.

Within minutes, the emergency services arrived. Quickly reacting to the situation, the technician checked Tom's vital signs. After quietly attaching the oxygen mask and programming the machine, the paramedics moved him into the waiting ambulance, shutting the door on Mary, her pale face still exhibiting a state of shock. As the ambulance left the drive, she got into her car to drive to the hospital.

By the time Tom arrived at the facility, he was partially revived. At the admissions area, the nurse approached Mary with a list of questions.

"Hi, I am Sarah, nurse in attendance to …"

Mary was very anxious but managed a weak smile. Wringing her hands, she interrupted with her own questions. "How is my husband? What went wrong? He was fine some hours back and … I did not look in on him, as he was busy completing a project …"

"Please calm down, Mrs. …"

"Call me Mary Carter, please … How is Tom?"

"Mr. Carter will be fine in some time. He was weak and exhausted. We decided to allow him to rest. In the meantime, I will need some basic information."

Sarah noted basic information about Tom on her data collection sheet:

- Age: fifty-one years
- Social security number …

Mary was tired and worried.

The nurse was a warm and understanding person. She was chirpy and quickly comforted Mary, handing her a mug with a freshly brewed coffee. "Mrs. Carter, you just need to relax a bit." Then she left the room.

A few minutes later, returning with initial reports, the nurse shared the results of the test. "His blood count is very low. That shows how anemic he is! We will be doing other tests and will bring you up to speed."

It was sometime later when the nurse took Mary to see Tom. Patting the leather couch, she added, "I think you would like to stay with him. I will stop by later with a pillow and some sheets."

Turning back, she said, "The cafeteria will close soon. If you want to get a snack, I can watch over Mr. Carter."

Mary responded with a tight smile, saying, "I'm fine."

She watched Tom's steady breathing and gradually got into a more comfortable position. *I need to keep alert. How did it happen? I was absolutely unaware that he had collapsed.*

Over the next few days, x-rays, blood tests, and twenty-four-hour urine tests revealed many new causes for concern. The tests showed the presence of serum protein, confirming the reason for Tom's anemic condition.

It took a protein electrophoresis to draw the conclusion that it was an abnormality in plasma cell formation, an unusually high number of white cells that were replicating fast. The bone marrow biopsy nailed the underlying causes as blood cancer known as multiple myeloma.

But the worst was yet to come.

Susan visited along with her husband. While the two of them were busy with the baby, Nurse Sarah entered with fresh update on Tom's health. "I'm afraid it's bad news … Your kidneys are severely damaged. You need immediate dialysis to sustain life."

Promising to come by sometime later, Nurse Sarah left Tom in a state of shock. He was devastated.

Opening his heart to Mary, he said, "It's almost like she has awarded me a death sentence! Oh, now what? It's just so sudden." Eyes brimming with unshed tears, shaking his head he said dejectedly, "I had no idea my life was heading this way. The end is so near!"

Mary held his hands. Looking into his eyes, she said reassuringly, "Tom, there are treatments available. Let's get them started. There's hope for survival. Please, let's explore …"

Then in her usual firm tone, she added, "And most certainly don't give up."

Talking to Mary magically changed Tom's mood.

Deep concern was visible in her transparent blue eyes; her grasp was warm, showing how much Tom meant to her. Her love and support brought new confidence and a sense of belonging to the middle-aged man, whose wrinkled eyes now carried love of life.

Susan was briefed on Tom's diagnosis. Her eyes were moist, but with effort she winked at her dad, smiling warmly and encouragingly. Mary, Susan, and Susan's husband watched Tom with bated breath, hoping he would decide quickly. There was worry that such a complicated disease would destroy him.

Tom, after saying a silent prayer, thought, *I still have enough life in me.*

The next morning Tom informed the doctor of his decision. Immediately he began his treatments. Special chemotherapy was scheduled, and he would start dialysis thrice a week, along with blood transfusions. Depending upon his body's response to therapy, a further course would be determined.

Tom hated dialysis and believed he had made an error in judgment by agreeing to undergo the procedure. With scrutiny he questioned the doctors. And being an optimist, he was sure that one day his normal kidney function would return.

Tom's hemoglobin levels improved, and his myeloma stabilized with treatment and erythropoietin. If only he did not need dialysis!

***

If it were possible to avoid dialysis, then many people with kidney disease would currently be living happily, free of such a hassle. Dialysis as a treatment is universally disliked. In 1943, Dr. Willem Kolff constructed the first dialysis machine. His mission to change things had begun when he helplessly watched a young man die of kidney failure. Stumbling upon an article published in 1913 on hemodialysis for animals, he was encouraged to explore further. Today dialysis is the first stage of treatment for people all over the world with kidney failure, as it effectively removes toxins accumulated in the bloodstream on account of poor kidney function. It is impossible to imagine how people with kidney disease could survive without some kind of dialysis being available.

Though Tom resented it, very soon he realized that dialysis was keeping him comfortable. Gradually he learned to carry on with this regimen.

Tom certainly had no way to control any of his health problems. Myeloma and dialysis had come accidently into his life. Mary watches him manage his life. She is grateful that his life was saved. The call to 911 was indeed made at the right time.

MANAGE OR YOU WILL WANE – ABBOTT STANLEY

Abbott Stanley lay uneasily on his bed, his eyes searching the ceiling for inspiration. It was clinic day. His hands crept downward, reaching to where his torso ended. Beyond that he had nothing more to touch. His lips twitched into a smile tinged with pain and sarcasm. The extent to which his body had been abused by the illness was unbelievable. In some time he would be assisted to dress and then he would leave.

On many a morning his thoughts would race back to the past, reliving those priceless moments. Every ounce of energy that flowed now came from memories of the distant past, which continued to bring him joy. His eyes would grow luminous with some sparks of life, and his lips would spread into a smile. Just for a few minutes he would give his deep hurt a break.

My childhood dreams and ambitions of becoming a surgeon, operating on people, and saving their lives—it happened just as I wanted. How glad I am for this chance. Many challenges came my way. I dared to face them, as other aspirants did. Finally that wonderful moment when I walked down the white hospital corridor arrived. The matron and duty nurse called out, "Welcome, Doctor," and congratulations poured from all quarters. The most wonderful party was thrown for me later that evening.

I was standing near the table laid with bouquets, dainty cupcakes, and a big spread of appetizers. Someone unscrewed a bottle of sparkling French Champagne. Dad and Mom were standing at a distance. As Deputy raised a glass for the toast, Dad and Mom found a way to come close to me. I turned to look at Dad. He wore a large smile and raised his glass for the toast. I saw Mom's eyes brim with tears of joy. How proud they felt. I felt good, real good. I knew that my ambitious streak, competitiveness, dedication, and hard work had paid off.

O my many years as a vascular surgeon performing complicated surgeries. It was always satisfying to see someone cured and return home to their family.

And, ah, those lectures I delivered. How much I loved it! Freshmen, medical graduate students, and trainees too—they gained knowledge on critical aspects of surgery. Showing my patients the value of personal targets in health care, publishing scientific papers—my own contributions to the medical world. I achieved it all, meeting my goals, performing up to my greatest potential. Life had been smooth sailing. It brought in loads of appreciation and a feeling of great achievement. What a glorious period that was! All the best moments were wrapped together.

Lots of work, lots of surgeries, many conferences, new breakthroughs. No time to sit and enjoy the moment. It was all lovely moments piled one on another. I wish I had taken a short holiday and spent time with Dad and Mom. How often Mom called and asked me to come, and I called last minute to cancel my visit. I made them sad. They knew I was busy. If only I had managed to see them more, then maybe things would be different.

And then that day, a warm sunny day, but yet I was shivering. A dark shrouded stranger met me as I left the clinic. I walked, and he followed at a distance. At home when I took my first sip of single malt, there was a knock on the door. I opened the door. Bowing, he introduced himself: "I am diabetes," he said, "and I am here to stay with you."

Abbott lay in his bed; the smile faded and was replaced by a distant look in his eyes, which were dark, glistening with pain and emotion. He recalled his reactions at that time.

How vehemently I refused to entertain the visitor. "It cannot be me" is what I said repeatedly. I am a learned surgeon. I know everything about health matters, my mind said. Later when the diagnosis was confirmed, how much it hurt to know that I had been caught unawares. I had to be reminded that diabetes is a silent and heartless disease—heartless because it changed my lifestyle. It restricted me from eating my favorite dishes. How very heartless!

When my patients learned to manage their illnesses and handle postoperative care as advised, it was very satisfying. Sometimes I felt remorse when the case was hopeless.

But in my own case, how did I not do it right? The truth hurts, and it hurts very bad!

My entry into rough seas with diabetes was a different experience. As reality sank in, I stepped into the shoes of the patient, with the gambit of periodic checking of blood sugar levels and giving myself insulin shots, while maintaining a busy career as a surgeon.

But it was late, very late, when I'd learned of my condition. I did my best, but slowly every door seemed to shut on me.

I was devastated as diabetes wreaked havoc with my body. My diminished eyesight affected my surgical skills. With peripheral circulatory disorder, my nervous system was badly affected and the feeling in my lower extremities was extremely reduced. I felt as if I were walking on cotton balls.

I had difficulty maintaining an erect posture over long periods. My autonomic system had been severely damaged. Poor blood circulation led to my losing first one leg and then the other. But I learned to manage with the prosthetic limb and, later on, the wheelchair!

Imagine, from a very active surgeon, I became a wheelchair-bound patient. Only my extensive reading brought me peace. Being sociable also helped. Unfortunately, my kidneys failed and I needed dialysis. Hemodialysis, dietary restrictions, and medications to control anemia, phosphorous, hemoglobin, blood pressure, and diabetes became part and parcel of my life.

I wish some complications had been arrested. I would be happier today if I'd had those chances.

Then with a smile brightening his face Abbott thought, But how can I forget those wonderful trips to meet friends! Yes, they were good. Getting out of Oregon was my real escape. Those were like adventures, away from this life strapped on the bed or to the wheelchair.

Today was different. Abbott spent more time analyzing his life than he had before. He became more questioning.

How did I manage all these debacles in life? Why did I let myself land from one stage to another? Is it possible that at times I was not compliant with diet and medication advice? I fooled myself into thinking that I did it well.

As problems kept piling on, I saw reason to go with the tide. Dread of dialysis evoked fear. I saw the possibility of a bleak end, but I stayed composed. To the best of my ability, I kept pace with the changes happening at each stage.

His eyes were moist with tears, and his insides hurt terribly. The unbearable pain shook his body all over. He showed little struggle to maintain himself … *No more of this,* he thought. His eyes were closed. His emotions took over and submerged him beneath the pressure of wretchedness. Soon the time to reminisce was past. Slowly his body collapsed. He took his last breath, now totally at peace.

Everyone remembered Abbott for his charming manners, determination, and sense of humor. Most importantly, people appreciated his forbearance. In him they saw acceptance of the disease and the determination to fight every stage of illness, an attitude to be emulated by patients arriving at this stage in their illness. In admiration the nephrologists, nurses, dietitian, social workers, and other professionals offered him encouragement and supported him emotionally.

***

The stages of illness, the pain, fear, and sorrow associated with it, was beyond everyone's capacity to endure.

But one can wonder what went through Abbott's mind as he helplessly let go of parts of his body. Did he accuse himself for being so naïve not to see diabetes coming? Early detection and timely action could have stalled the progression. After all, he advised his patients to be medically compliant. But now what? Losing body parts, fighting for survival, letting destiny shape his life when his fight failed—was it just too many things to handle?

What happened to Abbott could happen to you or me if we fail to understand the value of curbing our desire to splurge and thereby land ourselves into a health crisis. After all, isn't it all about living in moderation? Eat well, live right, see beyond just plain life, and achieve much more. Living life to the fullest need not be done with total abandon.

The story of this surgeon, however, shows something very remarkable.

After his death, society continued to respect him and recognize his surgical talents. A man who lost everything else retained his untarnished reputation. This shows the special place he held in a world that did not judge him as being a bad patient. His work determined his true position.

Thankfully he was not an object of pity. In the public mind, Abbott Stanley remains a man of great stature.

It is very common for people to be preoccupied with daily activities. The chance of ignoring one's health is high, as people tend to take health for granted. In this case, the doctor was so engrossed in caring for patients and placing great credence in their recovery that he never paused to wonder, *Am I eating properly? Am I feeling thirsty often?* He made other people's lives his priority. His wake-up call came too late. Thereafter, he struggled to catch up. That he missed the obvious signs of diabetes only shows his lost opportunity and fills a bag full of regrets. Abbott had people who respected him. But for a common man, such a health complication can draw flak from society. The world admires winners and ignores losers.

In the game of dice, the probability of a die falling to reveal all six dots at every throw is very low. The idea is far-fetched even for very deft sportsperson. The same is true for human beings: not everyone can be a winner. Life may become a dark road that has the potential to lighten up when an extraordinary power magically transforms the darkness. Not all lives are chosen for such a miraculous escapade. Respect for humanity, irrespective of faceup or facedown, must be our goal, leaving judgment to those empowered.

As we crawl toward the twilight of our lives, everything will become crystal clear. We will no longer think in terms of right or wrong, black or white, but will see life as gray in its simplest form. Truly there is never a winner or a loser; it is the statistical probability of a die falling faceup that seals one's fate.

PEOPLE TALK: CONTROL PHOSPHORUS – LUCY DREW

The middle-aged lady sat straight back in a chair by the window, her trembling fingers rolling the rosary beads as her lips moved soundlessly in worship. Her face was taut, her eyes glistening with unshed tears. Her mind was busy with thoughts.

It was about Lucy, her daughter, her child. She worried about Lucy all the time. How could she ever forget what a gruesome life Lucy had lived not too long ago?

The mother knew that tomorrow's sunrise would bring joyful showers of flowers. Champagne glasses would be raised by many family members and close friends, to toast for Lucy and Robert. Many people who would bless Lucy, as she was much loved.

The woman walked to the dresser to dab on some face powder and to tint her tired eyes that lacked luster because of the sleepless nights. *I should be happy and relaxed now. Why is my forehead wrinkled with worry? Why should I remember those bygone days when my most loved child, Lucy, faced a near-death situation? Why can I not love her and laugh with her today?* The mother questioned her silly behavior. But what could she do? Those memories were still so strong and fresh.

She remembered that day very well. It came back in a flash.

It was the great countdown to the millennium. The world had been positioned to believe that even the sun's glory would change. Some imaginary wheels would move everyone physically from the twentieth to the twenty-first century. Euphoria and excitement drove new concepts for party planning the world over. It was not simply another year-end party.

The Canton household always partied in style. They got ready to celebrate the turn of the century with great fanfare. So adept were they in doing things with aplomb. They had the barbeque aflame, grilling thick, juicy steaks; the bar open with glasses waiting to be filled, liquor bottles stacked neatly, and chilled wine and beer left refrigerated; and tables laid with large platters of grilled vegetables, small chicken tarts, burgers, chips, cheese, and crackers, all plated, to please different palates.

The plan was to keep the dance floor hopping until late at night, with alcohol freely flowing, until everyone was ready to drop. Speculations were rife, with many saying that the year 2000 would break all barriers economically and socially. The world would be a great place to exist.

Guests came in, leaving a trail of mixed fragrances. But Lucy, who was fully keyed into the celebration, was showing signs of fatigue and discomfort, which she couldn't understand. But she decided to remain cheerful and let her hair down, dancing to the blaring music. A few hours later, much before midnight, she felt she would collapse. She retired quietly to her room. She would rest a little.

It was the morning rays of the sun that stirred her from her deep slumber. But Lucy was still feeling odd, uneasy.

Her parents were concerned that Lucy had retired early the night before while guests were asking for her. Seeing her under the weather, her mother rushed her to the clinic. The senior doctor began tests, starting with blood pressure.

"I find your high blood pressure is high. We need to do some more tests. In the meantime, you must start on some medicines to control your blood pressure." The doctor started a battery of tests. These revealed chronic kidney disease caused by hypertension. Lucy was put on health alert. Diet and medications were advised, along with dialysis. In sync with her attitude and lifestyle, she opted for peritoneal dialysis (PD).

Lucy continued to enjoy life within the limits placed on her by her health condition.

But something happened to bring her joy to an abrupt end. Peritonitis inflamed her abdominal wall, and she was hospitalized. Under expert care, she recovered after a course of antibiotic therapy. Her health restored, she bounced back into her life routine with her PD. This was a phase in which she was less stressed about her health.

As she watched with love and concern, Lucy's mother's stomach curled with tension. When Lucy was finished with the routine hospital visits, she quickly settled back into her PD routine. She seemed happy.

What will happen to Lucy? Is my worry well-founded? She thought, *A mother's heart always knows!* She smiled, sad at her own rightness. She hoped she would be proved wrong.

***

It happens all the time. People under extreme stress indulge in food. Being a foodie for a person with normal health may result in obesity, but the life of a kidney patient who is a food becomes compromised. There is a food chart to follow indicating a recommended daily consumption of products with phosphorus, potassium, and sodium. If the balance is disturbed, the consequence is beyond imagination.

Lucy's phosphorus levels rose high, confirmed by repeated blood evaluations. Much to her caretaker's consternation, she refused to take the warning signals seriously.

On account of her high blood phosphorous level, she suffered from common cardiovascular complications. Peritoneal dialysis, even if done daily, is poor at removing phosphorous from the body. Lucy was forced to change her diet by reducing phosphorus intake. Additional phosphorus binders were introduced to bind phosphorus in her gut so that her body would not absorb the phosphorus.

But these measures were insufficient or late in coming. The fangs of hypophosphatemia and secondary hyperparathyroidism in their severe forms caught her. Doctors smoothed her ruffled feathers by saying, "This is recognized worldwide as most likely among dialysis patients."

Lucy slowly developed other complications including an enlarged heart with poor function. The doctors inserted a defibrillator to prevent irregular heart rhythm and low blood pressure, but the device infected her heart. Miraculously, after the device was removed, she got relief from antibiotic therapy.

The condition of her parathyroid glands had deteriorated, so most of them were removed during a clinical procedure called parathyroidectomy.

Over the course of many years of changing lanes from a high number of medical challenges, to a stable life, to another health calamity, Lucy's attitude toward life underwent a change. Through the heavy clouds covering her, she saw some light penetrate, which gave her a reason to smile.

In 2004, Lucy Canton received the most precious gift of her life: a kidney transplant.

Now her mother thought that she should focus on the upcoming event, the thing that needed to be recorded as most memorable, namely, the wedding that would unite Lucy with Robert. *I shouldn't be vulnerable to sad thoughts,* she kept reminding herself.

She had watched Lucy while the veil was being placed firmly on her head and had felt her heart flowing with happiness. At the church, with her excitement increasing the pace of her heartbeat, she had stood mesmerized upon seeing Lucy looking enthralled with happiness. She experienced a unique moment of happiness. She wiped a tear away and prayed for happy times for Lucy and Robert.

Time went by. Lucy came home to visit less often. The mother reprimanded herself: *I must realize Lucy has new responsibilities, including a husband to care for.* She thought of the dark days of the past sometimes with sadness, and at other times she sent a silent prayer upward.

And then one day over lunch she reminded Lucy of her follow-up tests. Lucy smiled. "Oh yes, I must do that. I will do it soon, Mom!" But judging from Lucy's tone, her mother was not convinced of her daughter's earnestness.

The next morning, Lucy's mother took her window seat. The beads between her fingers were moving slowly now, as her heart was submerged in a familiar fear.

A few months later, her fear became a reality.

Lucy had lost her kidney. Time for worry began. Now things were serious.

***

Families with kidney patients also go through the ordeals of the disease. Without actually experiencing dialysis or the massive implications of a transplant, parents are aware of the agony and feel sad for the pain experienced by their son or daughter. It may be simply watching the child endure the pricks of a needle, seeing large volumes of blood circulating in the dialyzer, and wondering what it feels like to have the water, blood, and other fluids moving around, disturbing their child's peace. It's seeing the person's frown and expression of frustration and trying to fathom the extent of the sorrow. Lucy's mother, a dedicated caregiver, was extremely sensitive to even a feather touch on Lucy.

Kidney transplants give people the opportunity to lead normal lives. But it is a package deal. With the new kidney, new responsibilities need to be shouldered. There's simply no way to take it lightly. The body shows symptoms early enough. One needs to catch these signs and get back to the doctor and clinic immediately.

Sadly for Lucy, it was too late. Very soon after her wedding, she began dialysis.

WHAT'S IN YOUR RED BAG? – RYAN GRIFFITH, UNITED KINGDOM

RG. That's what friends called him, and he loved it.

He was having an evening birthday dinner, and he had a Facebook friend asking him many questions.

"By the way, what city are you from?"

"I'm from the UK, not from the US!" RG said teasingly.

"RG, tell me a little about your health."

"Oh, my health is a great secret. I need time to explain all the medical terms. You need to understand and appreciate my experience."

"I think, RG, you're being very possessive and want to hold tight."

He used the laugh emoji and said, "Later, tomorrow." He could see his wife was ready. If he didn't get up to go now, they would be late.

"See you later, GS." Though she had a beautiful name, RG chose to call her by her initials.

As he and his wife rode to the party, RG's mind went back to the conversation. *What should I talk about? Is GS going to understand all the different things I have in my bag?*

His wife saw him deep in thought and nudged her seventy-year-old husband. Without a preamble, RG began talking as if continuing an old conversation. "Remember how I was shocked by that collapse almost four decades back? I can't stop wondering why on earth it happened!"

RG and his wife, having arrived at their destination, held hands as they walked into the party room. The evening was interesting. RG relaxed and mingled.

Late that night, after the party, RG pulled out the red bag and reached in it for the files. One was from 1972, embossed with his merchant navy company's name and emblem. It had a sticker that read, "Accident."

He read the report out loud: "'On duty, a nasty accident with a four-ton steel block, landing on his back. The initial x-rays showed mild lumbar fracture. Patient was able to walk when discharged. Heavy doses of painkillers have settled him.'

"That's their summation. But what happened next showed no evidence of connection to the accident.

"And … the painkillers stayed with me." He smiled sadly.

The second file was from 1986. It was marked "Occupational Asthma."

RG read the report, softly now, as it was well after midnight and he didn't want to disturb his wife. "'It is an occupational lung disease, a kind of asthma. There's inflammation in the airway, reversible airway obstruction, and bronchospasm. It may be due to environment at workplace.

"'Rx – symptoms include coughing, wheezing, shortness of breath, and some tightness in the chest area. Some mild nasal involvement seems to be present.'"

He remembers how angry he'd been about this. Were the two events connected, the accident and then the occupational asthma, which actually might be the result of the accident? Nobody had come up with this theory.

Then he picked up the 1993 file. "Hiatal hernia," he read in a tired voice.

Another lousy one! More of a nuisance! Slowly opening the file, he read what he had scribbled on the inner flap: "An inner body part pushed itself and occupied some other area, giving rise to a hiatal hernia."

Then he read the report: "'Observed an opening in the diaphragm separating the esophagus from the chest. The esophagus passing through the hiatus has connected to the stomach. The stomach is pushing toward the chest.

"'Rx – Proton pump inhibitors (PPIs) prescribed to reduce the acid in the stomach.'"

PPIs are commonly used to treat acid reflux, stomach ulcers and the part of the gut called the duodenum. Most people who take a PPI do not develop any side effects.

"Another journey of sorts now began, with more medications piling on my counter!" he said, amused.

"Ah, there it is. The secret one I was thinking about while chatting with GS."

Pulling it out of the bag, his eye caught the big red "???" on the cover. His forefinger ran over the figure. He drew a deep breath.

"What a great letdown! Suddenly I discovered that my kidneys were losing their function and I had chronic kidney disease. Apparently my doctors didn't feel too concerned, as they never spoke about it."

RG's eyes grew moist with tears. His mind went through the past events. *They noticed and didn't tell me, or they never really studied my report in detail to notice it. Was I too busy or I too much pain not to see where my health was going?*

Wiping his eyes, he reprimanded himself. "Why hurt when nothing is reversible in life!"

After five minutes of sitting quietly and taking charge of his emotions, he picked up the last file.

In 2015 his health had gone downhill. He was rushed to the hospital with an emergent condition. Many tests were done over the next few days, and finally multiple myeloma (cancer of the plasma cells) and chronic lymphocytic leukemia (blood and bone marrow cancer) were both detected. Immediately the doctors scheduled several cycles of chemotherapy.

Between the cycles, RG developed a heart problem. Right in the midst of his confused state of health, he underwent a double heart stent operation.

Finally the chemotherapy came to an end.

Heaving a sigh of relief, RG had smiled and suggested to his wife, "I've had enough drama and could do with a holiday!"

Apparently loving the idea, she had spread her arms out.

But the doctors somehow had extraordinary energy and they suggested a stem cell transplant as the next treatment for remission.

Recalling what happened next, RG said, "How despairing it was! My nephrologist denied the treatment, saying that with my kidney condition it was not appropriate."

An accidental discovery of chronic kidney disease (CKD) and the rejection of a stem cell transplant was a sad culmination, showing how deeply CKD could impact a person's life.

Ryan Griffith's red bag got its contents purely by accident. One condition seems to have led to another, and all of them were beyond any mathematical calculation! In the 1970s medical prescriptions were different. Long-term use of medications is said to cause CKD. So the numerous files all found their mysterious way into one bag.

MARIA'S BABY WAS SAVED! – MARIA ROMANO

Changes in the life of twenty-two-year-old Maria Romano seemed constant. But after a long time, one certain change made her very happy. As she tried to overcome the emotional moment with tears flowing down her beautiful cheeks, her right hand gently pressed her abdomen, looking for a lightning connection with the little one residing there. Her lips parted softly, calling out, "Sweetheart."

Hendric Romano wove his arms through her arms to hold her close to him. He knew this was the ultimate joy of their life. He brushed her cheeks gently, wiping away traces of tears, and the two of them laughed in happiness.

Slowly they walked toward their car. "Where shall we celebrate?"

Maria's eyes shone brightly as she said, "Brunch Place." Let's enjoy our usual Sunday brunch in advance."

Hendric started his car. He whistled softly through the ride. Suddenly his brow creased and his eyes grew grave. An hour later he and his wife would go to the dialysis center. That was Maria's thrice-a-week routine. Today it would be difficult! Maria would suddenly be facing the whole truth. So happiness was this ride, the brunch, and …

Maria was chattering away. "So unexpected this is! I never dreamed of this!" She talked of the baby and how they needed to do detailed planning. Her excitement was infectious. Hendric joined in the conversation, trying to keep the upbeat mood.

But it was when Maria began dialysis that she faced reality.

"Am I allowed this? For a kidney patient, getting pregnant could cause complications! Should I have talked to my nephrologist beforehand?"

Slowly nervousness set in. After an hour or so, sadness crept in and she was sobbing softly. The attending nurse noticed this and paged the psychologist.

The elderly matron-type psychologist walked down the hallway and called out to Maria. Maria's agitated face tried a smile. The matron took a chair for a chat. "Is everything all right, Maria?" she asked gently.

With some effort and prompting, Maria shared her latest news. Soon the nurse and technicians stopped by to congratulate her. Slowly she regained her composure.

A few days later she met her nephrologist.

Opening her file, the doctor read, "'Twenty-two years old, developed chronic kidney disease secondary to IgA nephropathy. Has had irregular menstrual periods.'

"So, young lady, now your pregnancy report confirms it." He looked up, smiling. Then reaching out to lightly pat her shoulder, he said, "Let's handle it properly. It is important to watch your vitals and be careful with medications so you have an easy delivery."

Over the next few months, Maria was scheduled for extra dialysis treatments. Her fluid balance was monitored; her blood pressure was watched and treated; and her anemia was corrected with intravenous iron and erythropoietin therapy. The pregnancy was full term and she delivered with a C-section.

"I always told you pregnancy is safe if well managed. It simply needs close monitoring. You're a good patient." The nephrologist's tribute brought a smile to her tired lips.

"Thank you so much, Doctor. You protected my child!"

***

In Maria's case, talking to her doctor made her pregnancy easy. Good and continuous health monitoring saved the baby. Pregnancy for patients who have IgA nephropathy is considered to be high risk, as high or low blood pressure or anemic conditions could affect the baby's development. The patient needs to work closely with the nephrologists and comply with the medical advice and directions given.

I'LL STAY ON DIALYSIS – RUTH REAGAN

The doctor was studying the annual test results of a twenty-year-old, Ruth Reagan. He remembered her from the previous visit as a happy and fun-loving person. She would be the last patient that evening.

With a soft knock, Ruth entered through the door. With a smile, the doctor greeted her. Starting the conversation, he asked, "How are you?"

Ruth smiled and responded with honesty: "Doctor, I am well, but I am tired after a long day at school."

The doctor smiled and continued, "I am sure. But, Ruth, I have here results of the blood test. There is a reason why you are slowing down. Your high blood pressure is a worry, and your kidneys are functioning poorly. Your kidney function could deteriorate with the passage of time."

With a sinking heart, Ruth listened to him talk about aggressively controlling her blood pressure to preserve her kidney function, making significant changes to her lifestyle, becoming more active physically, observing dietary limitations, and adhering to a medication regimen to control blood pressure. She decided to do it all.

Four years later, dialysis became necessary to sustain life. Ruth understood the merits of both peritoneal and hemodialysis treatment and which of these was an effective therapy for failed kidneys. She preferred to receive hemodialysis in-center three times a week, three to four hours each time. Ruth needed a dialysis shunt placed in her arm for dialysis treatment.

Through this period Ruth stood determined, choosing to receive treatment as opposed to not receiving treatment. She accepted the significant limitations in her lifestyle as opposed to inviting death. She desired to live no matter what.

In Ruth's words, "I faced my share of dialysis and non-dialysis-related complications. Sometimes it was revisions of dialysis shunts, suddenly shots of pain from a severe bone disease, abnormal heartbeats, even facial paralysis. But my twenty years into dialysis with reasonably stable condition is encouraging." As an afterthought she added, "I will never consider trading my current condition with the other alternative. In fact I am now promoting this treatment for the stable life for a kidney patient."

Though transplant is an option offered to many people based on their chance of a good life post-transplant and if chance of recurrence of the disease is not likely, people who are medically unfit for a transplant must choose to remain positive even on dialysis.

Ruth was very happy to remain on dialysis, for personal reasons.

Many people make such a choice because they do not want anyone to sacrifice a kidney to save them, or else they are afraid of having to face a failed transplant. Handling the many aspects of kidney disease takes plenty of courage and an ability to withstand pressures and fight against all odds. At every stage the disease keeps a person actively involved in health care. Neglecting any aspect at any stage is playing with fire. In the early stages of kidney disease, with proper diet and medications, kidney failure can be postponed for several decades. While on dialysis, many danger zones emerge, as will be seen from many narratives in *Who Lives, Who Dies with Kidney Disease*. Life after a transplant brings with it management issues.

After all, this disease is for a lifetime.

FEAR OF THE WHITE COAT – SUBODH MUKHERJEE

Subodh Mukherjee studied the laboratory report as he walked out of the clinic. The high level of creatinine caught his eye. It was 2.0 mg/dL, when the normal range of creatinine is 0.6–1.2 mg/dL.

Now what's going on? he wondered, a little worried about this rise. He'd met his physician, Dr. Lal, who suggested that he see a nephrologist. It was a disturbing thought.

In 1991, during a medical test, Subhodh had been alerted about his blood pressure being very high. It was in the range of 180/100. The same doctor had prescribed him blood pressure medication, which he had religiously taken for several years. Fear of any further health-related news had made him compliant with his medication regimen. Without going back to the doctor, he had managed to renew his prescriptions without much problem.

Married to Moushmi, and with his kids very young, Subodh believed he had managed his health well and with responsibility.

But now in 1999, as he turned forty years old, things seemed to have changed. This blood test report was a shocker! The Indian doctor had also hinted that he'd lost 50 percent of his kidney function.

That evening over a cup of tea, he shared his concerns with Moushmi. "There's some problem … Remember the blood test I did? So … there's protein in the blood. My creatinine level is going up, and Dr. Lal has said almost 50 percent of the kidney function is gone!"

"What? Kidney failure?" she shouted, as if she'd been hit by a rock.

"Not yet, but it will happen in time."

"What does Dr. Lal want you to do?"

"Go to a nephrologist, a kidney specialist!"

Moushmi sat still. She knew it was a tough situation. Subodh had a phobia of going to doctors and hospitals. He would joke with her, "I suffer from white coat syndrome!"

She was worried for her family.

In August 2003, Subodh's legs were swollen, so when he went to the doctor, a blood test revealed that his creatinine had risen to 8 mg/dL. For a better lifestyle, he was put on peritoneal dialysis (PD). The surgery for placing the catheter in the peritoneum cavity presented a problem, so a second surgery was needed.

PD worked well for Subodh, but he had some very unusual experiences.

In December 2005, he went with his family to India to attend a family wedding. Once he had fixed his seat belt, the metal buckle was accidentally resting on top of the catheter's exit site. This pressure caused the cusp to leak.

Such an incident is avoidable, but when it happens it causes panic and can make a person feel very unsure of life. Getting back to the doctor to change the catheter was critical. It was not that Subodh didn't learn from his mistake, but when he had another incident he was terrified.

In November 2008, while Subodh was on the treadmill with 1000 cc of fluid dialysate, the bouncing of the fluid caused the exit site to leak. The leak continued for some time, leading to severe peritonitis. This meant that his catheter needed to be replaced. For some time he had to stay on hemodialysis. Both these episodes showed how easy it is for a person on PD to take things for granted and become complacent. Subodh felt these situations could have been avoided.

Moushmi had said, "Maybe you should have opted for the transplant when the call came in 2005!"

Subodh could not remind her of his concern for their children's education. They were still in school. So he sought a postponement. But he knew that it was the best decision for him.

Finally, January 2009 brought about a change to his life. He had his transplant.

His own assessment on his health is as follows:

> My first test, in 1991, showed high blood pressure [BP]. Thereafter, I went to get medication refills from the pharmacy without checking my blood pressure.
>
> I should have done periodical blood tests and monitored my blood pressure.
>
> In 1999 when Dr. Lal suggested I meet a nephrologist, I should have followed his advice. The nephrologist may have changed my medicines and even increased dosage to keep my BP under control.
>
> I was comfortable with the refills, which meant not meeting a doctor. Fear of meeting a doctor who would tell me about my serious health condition made me lose my kidney. Having a limited vision of life and the belief that I could live life on my own terms was my tragic downfall. With great humility I have understood that one must open doors to wisdom and never allow fear to manage one's life.
>
> The belt's buckle damaging my dialysis catheter, and exercising on a treadmill that affected the catheter's exit site due to the abdomen's muscle movement, seem too small to think about. These so-called small mistakes in reality cost so much pain and resulted in so many unwanted complications. In dialysis both big and small things need to be understood and taken into consideration.

FORTY-SEVEN YEARS OF VALUABLE DIALYSIS EXPERIENCE – THOMAS LEHN, GERMANY

Today, I, Thomas Lehn, can say I'm the longest-living survivor on hemodialysis in the whole world. There is no pride in living so long with this treatment, but to stand as a testimony to medical advancements makes me wonder at the Lord for choosing for me this life.

I recall clearly, I had just turned fourteen years old and I faced shocking experiences with regard to my health and life. I want to share with you an abstract of the worst time of my life, including episodes that I can clearly remember, even today.

On August 20, 1970, I was deathly sick, temporarily disoriented, and blind, with extraordinarily high blood pressure. My small body was filled with over ten liters of water. I lay in the intensive care unit of the surgical clinic in Heidelberg. The late Dr. Hans Wolf Schueler, a physician and urologist, held my hand. He checked my left hand first, and then my right arm, searching for blood vessels. For several minutes, with great concentration, he closed his eyes. Then he declared that I would not die from the uremic toxins and the fluids in my body. He would put me into emergency surgery as soon as possible to fix a Scribner shunt.

This became the first step for my first dialysis.

Photo 1

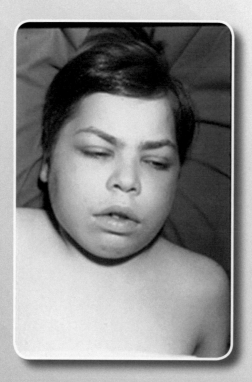

My condition being so bad, I couldn't see him, but I could hear him say, "Chin up, my boy. We will manage this. We will be set you up with this. Please be brave. You will live!"

Dead or Alive

It was the early rays of the sun that woke me. I stretched my body and felt constricted. Looking around, I saw some tubes and the walls—white walls. I remembered having been put in a hospital after being diagnosed with terminal kidney insufficiency. It had seemed as if I was awarded a death sentence. During the 1970s, dialysis was not so advanced and few people were lucky to get treated. (Today, in developing countries and economically poor countries, patients still face such conditions and feel insecure.)

Many things were wrong. I was young, I was far away from family, and I suffered multiple morbid conditions. I felt more dead than alive! For many days I was in the small room of the university surgical clinic at Heidelberg, and in that room also was at an infernal dialysis machine. I can't remember how many days and nights I was on dialysis. It is possible that I'd been able to survive twelve hours of dialysis only because of Valium. I never noticed when another kid next to me had dialysis and either fought for life or succumbed to death. That was the bitter choice: death or life!

I recall there were two dialysis units. Even in those days, there were ten children below fourteen years of age receiving dialysis there. So with a round-the-clock shift, the kids took turns receiving dialysis. Sadly a new kid was admitted to the dialysis program only when a space opened up or when another patient died. Sometimes I sit and wonder how the doctors and nurses worked so hard with that type of mental stress. It is true about the first few hours of admission.

After three sessions of dialysis, I felt better. By now, about eight liters of fluid and the high concentration of the uremic substances had been removed from my body. Surprisingly all this was done by a rustic Travenol dialysis machine, which stands as no comparison to today's advanced and more effective dialyzers.

And then, yes, my eyes could see my mother again. She visited me every day.

Photo 2

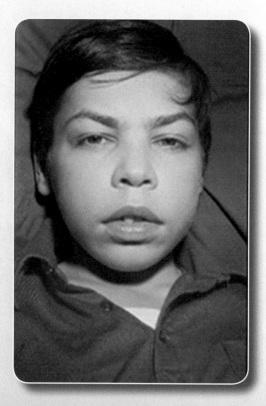

After twelve hours of dialysis, I wasn't able to walk upright for the first few hours. The next day I would rest. I was mostly very ill, so I was taken to the children's hospital by ambulance. Sometimes I woke up in an emergency room and would go later back to the children's hospital.

Childhood Dialysis—a Big Experience

Today everyone talks of complications. Back then nobody knew what kind of long-term complications could be expected in children. They knew that in relation to adult patients, children have unstable blood vessels. Would the young organism tolerate the strenuous hemodialysis duration? How would young patients grow up? Did dialysis affect the metabolism and hormone levels in children? Would the dialysis filter away hormones, especially growth hormones? Would children enter puberty? Would they be able to lead independent lives in the future? Would they be able to have a normal education and pursue a career along with getting dialysis treatment? Was the Scribner shunt a permanent connection for hemodialysis? What problems could occur in the long term? Was it possible to live a normal life with transplantation?

Photo 3

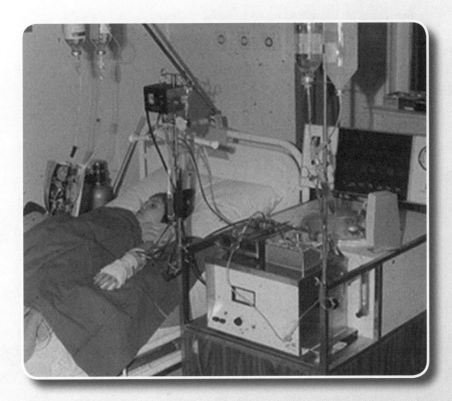

There were thousands of questions, but nobody knew the answers at that time. It was quite the learning experience.

Better Technology, Shorter Dialysis Time
Over time, the dialysis machines grew better and were lifesavers.

New dialyzers called "capillary artificial kidneys" were developed. They cleaned the blood better and faster. Another good development came with the 2008S from Fresenius, which had ultrafiltration. This new machine with high-volume ultrafiltration helped prevent many health problems to bring patients comfort and ease. It could calibrate weight gained and lost. The standard machine included a heparin pump that could help you control the Fragmin or heparin. Bicarbonate dialysis treatment was better and gentle than the acetate dialysis known previously. The Gambro AK5, as it was called, was the most modern dialysis machine with good electronic features. This freed up the dialysis staff to care for others who needed care. Alarms were triggered if there was something wrong with the machine's working condition or the patient was in any danger. The dialysis schedule was reduced to twice a week for ten hours each time, and then to three times per week, eight hours each time.

From Tommy to Thomas
During the years, I used my dialysis time trying to understand the medical and technical advancements in dialysis and gathering medical knowledge. My thirst for knowledge about my illness made me question doctors and nurses, who were really very helpful. I depended on them for information, as Internet was nonexistent.

I got my education with teachers' help as a guest student in the local school. I successfully completed my education, with a high school leaving certificate. My youth was not much different from that of my healthy young friends.

In 1975 I met my Beate. We fell in love. In 1978 I was trained to be a computer programmer. In October 1980 I took my job. I am still in employment there. For thirty-seven years I have been employed as a systems engineer.

Photo 4

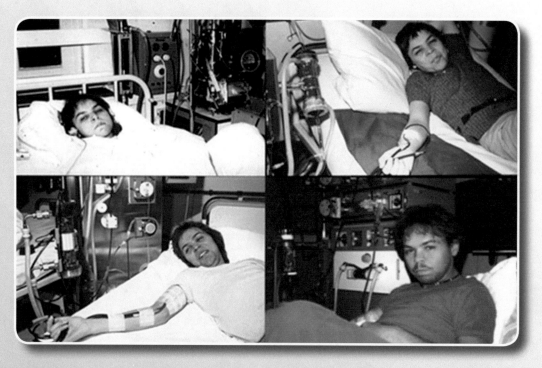

Home Hemodialysis

In 1983 I began to receive home hemodialysis. In 1984 Beate and I got married.

I decided against the transplant, because I discovered home hemodialysis to be the perfect treatment. It was, for me, the most suitable renal replacement therapy.

Photo 5

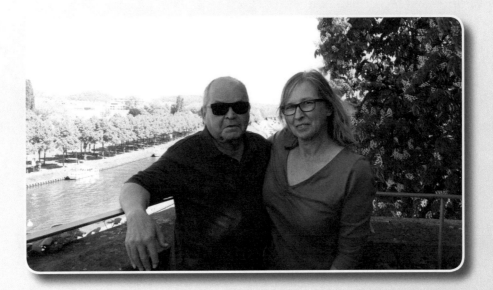

Thomas Lehn
Bergstrasse 30
55218 Ingelheim
Germany
On the internet: http://www.thomas-lehn.de or http://www.dialyseshunt.com
Email: Thomas.Lehn@online.de

Travel and Dialysis Worldwide

Beate and I love to travel, and we've stayed at many places all over the world with dialysis treatment. Today it is possible to go on dialysis holidays all over the world. We have been to Egypt, Turkey, South Africa, the USA, the Dominican Republic, Greece, Mexico, Jamaica, Canary Islands, and Croatia, among other places.

Photo 6

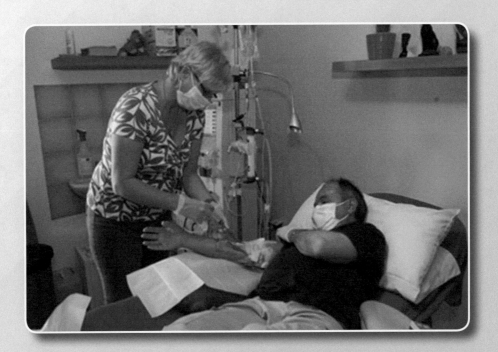

Kidney Transplant—Not My Cup of Tea

In early years I evaluated transplant options. Some health issues gave me reason to avoid transplant. By choosing home dialysis, I grew more comfortable. Over the years my views on kidney transplant changed.

My opinion is that when my body will accept a foreign organ only with the use of medications called immunosuppressants, which can decrease the immune system's defensive capabilities, and when my body will continue to fight that organ all my life, preventing it from being considered as part of my body, is a sad situation. In addition, the transplanted organ is always subject to renal failure. The immunosuppressive agents in the body set into motion autonomous processes over which neither medicine nor I have any control. This fact makes me uncomfortable.

I am not against transplantation, but I will accept it only if all possible components of a transplant are clarified. And, no, I'm not registered for a kidney transplant.

How Do I Manage?

I know that my health has been managed by paying attention to certain rules. I am certain that when I refuse foods with high levels of phosphates and potassium, I'm fine. When I don't drink so much and I take my prescribed medications (vitamin D, a phosphate binder, and so on), I am fine. If I follow my long dialysis routine of six hours or more, sticking to a frequency of three to four times a week, I'll be fine. For me it is very important to have good medical consultants. I also want to be properly informed. My social environment is important too. Family and friends need to accept that dialysis comes with baggage, including additional diseases. With all these components and compromises, my cooperative wife and I try to lead an almost normal life—hoping it will last for a long, long time.

My Basket of Complications

In forty-seven-odd years I have seen many problems, and at times my health has been touch-and-go. It matters to me, but I know that grab baskets sometimes contain things not of our choice. My bones have been damaged by the long-term dialysis, which is based on the chemical process of calcium phosphate metabolism in the kidney. I often have bone pain and joint pain. My parathyroid glands were removed twenty-eight years ago. Five years back I had carpal tunnel syndrome surgery on both hands. Sometimes I experience neuropathy in the legs and amyloidosis in the right foot, both of which are fairly predictable, but not to be underestimated. I am satisfied with my health, and I hope that I can maintain my condition.

My life motto: *Life is strong but beautiful!* Live your dreams as long as you can.

COMPLICATIONS WITH LUPUS – SALINA GABRIEL

Salina cried out in anguish, "Mom, why is this pain in my joints not subsiding? It tires me so much. And this skin rash all over the body also bothers me. What's gone wrong with me?"

Her mother examined the rash and was worried about the rapid spread. She knew of some good local remedies that were available, so she purchased some for Salina's use.

But the rash was so adamant that it continued to show on Salina's skin, leaving her unhappy.

In 1983, Salina Gabriel was a carefree sixteen-year-old who pursued her education, enjoyed life with her family, and did all the fun things that people do in their youth. But when she suffered from this joint pain, which was in her hands and her upper and lower extremities, she was depressed. She ached all the time! She tired easily. She struggled to perform normal routine activities, whereas her friends were bursting with energy and liveliness.

"Mom, what's happening? I feel so very lousy! I have lost ninety-eight pounds in just a few months. How can there be so much happening?" she said, breaking down under the enormous weight of this unknown disease.

Her mother had noticed her weight reduction. Salina's skeletal look had bothered her too.

Gradually other things piled up. Salina was bothered about her lack of appetite and her low energy level, which sometimes make it impossible for her even to feed herself. And then the blood test showed her nutrition levels dropped lower than required for a healthy body. Local remedies failed to revive her health, and suddenly it dawned on mother and daughter alike that Salina's deteriorated condition would need medical attention.

The doctor immediately hospitalized her. Salina went into a coma, remaining in that state for three days. In the intensive care unit, she was hooked up to heart-monitoring equipment. Her large family and friends were worried. They prayed fervently, showing their support and visiting her in the hospital. Her boyfriend suffered from uncontrollable pangs of sorrow at seeing Salina in such a critical condition.

When Salina came out of the coma, the attendant doctor disclosed the results of all the tests. She had lupus, an autoimmune disease that could become very dangerous. The doctor explained the disease and the line of treatment, involving some powerful medications to control the disease. Though these drugs had serious side effects, they were essential for treating the disease and preventing its progression.

After a two-month stay in the hospital, with the best of treatment from the doctors, Salina was back on her feet. But for the next three years, Salina was occupied with fighting the disease. She was tormented with a low blood count, aching joints, a facial rash, high blood pressure, fevers, muscle pain, hair loss, mouth ulcers, and fatigue.

For a teenager it was tough to handle all these miseries. In her depressed state, Salina frequently fought the temptation to commit suicide. To add to the complications, she developed salmonella infection after consuming some snake pills from a local pharmacy.

Soon her kidneys showed signs of failing. Treatments were started, with chemotherapy being the first line of treatment. But Salina was unable to tolerate any more than three sessions of chemotherapy. In time, when her levels of creatinine rose high and her kidneys failed, she began dialysis.

After a year and eight months, Salina received her twin sister's kidney so that she would not become dialysis dependent and would enjoy a reasonably good life. But through this new phase of life, Salina was concerned about her sister's well-being.

The kidney transplant was successful. Salina took her medications religiously, though her face looked like a chipmunk's. She wanted to care for her prized kidney. She got married. Within four years of the kidney transplant, she had a baby girl. By now Salina had gotten used to a reasonably comfortable life. Her lupus was in remission. Her sister was also in good health.

But in Salina's life, things were never peaceful. Three years later she was divorced, and a month after that she was diagnosed with cancer of the vulva. After nearly twenty-five biopsies, of which five revealed she had cancer, and the need to undergo three extensive surgeries was established, the oncologists were advising removal of the cancerous growth.

Twelve years later Salina is grateful for being free of cancer.

After having lived seventeen years with the transplanted kidney, she chose to stop her immunosuppressant medication. Her daughter, now a teenager, is her source of joy. Salina continuous fighting stress and depression, which surfaces now and then.

***

Lupus is such a rare autoimmune disease that people are overwhelmed by the unexpected ways in which it impacts health. The fact that it can flare up anytime and sometimes lead to multiple organ failure keeps people on tenterhooks. Living with lupus is tough, but medical advancements have made survival a reality in cases where there is an opportunity to get treatment and manage the many conditions arising as a result of the disease.

DIABETES PLAYED TRUANT – JOSÉ THOMAS

José Thomas sat in the restaurant. He had ordered a small meal. Many things were not permitted now with his restricted diet. Twelve years ago, at this same place, he had met her. He sat back and reminisced.

The music floated around the fully occupied restaurant. People ordered their meals and chatted mostly. At the far end, she was dipping into her favorite, garlic chicken pasta, sipping wine, and enjoying the soulful music. José, the lead singer, was a jubilant young man. His band played at several restaurants upon special invitation. He made it a point to go around and chat with people after the session. This gave the evening a certain warmth, and was much appreciated by the regulars at the joint.

The applause was loud as he completed the last song for the evening.

"Thank you, friends, for being such a great audience," José said, waving both arms alternatively.

Though he was overweight, he was a happy man, content with life and his music.

José recalled that evening. "I remember that kind lady was sitting at this very table. She had praised me for my wonderful spirit." Then, shrugging his shoulders, he sat and sipped water, wondering what his future would be. "My wonderful life was simply cut short. It just came tumbling down," he murmured, as if in a trance.

He chuckled at the unanticipated changes that had happened in his life.

It all had begun with a few conditions that didn't seem serious at all. He had faced fatigue, which even after a good night's sleep didn't seem to vanish. Friends had asked him to lose weight and do strenuous exercise. But being so overweight meant that even starting any exercise was a humungous task!

When he had grown irritated with his general health, he had seen a doctor. After a few preliminary checkups, he was directed to a laboratory for a few blood tests. He was diagnosed with type 2 diabetes, which grew into the much dreaded kidney failure.

This setback had come with several responsibilities. Now he needed to be on regular dialysis, follow dietary restrictions, and learn how to maintain a reasonable lifestyle.

All these things went smoothly for a brief spell. José's health continued to deteriorate, though. With peripheral neuropathy and vascular disease setting in, it became difficult for him to perform normal activities. So in many aspects, his output was significantly limited. The greatest misfortune was the stroke, which affected his speech, threatening his professional life. José felt very demoralized and depressed.

Smaller irritants with his dialysis shunt had meant multiple revisions to make it functional. The effects of peripheral vascular disease took their toll. He had to undergo amputation of part of the index fingers of his right hands and all the toes of his left foot because of poor circulation and onset of gangrene.

These complications were accompanied by pain, infection of his lower extremities, frequent hospitalizations, and visits to orthopedists and other specialists. Life changed dramatically; he could not drive to dialysis, and he lost control over his health.

José knew in his heart that without the support of his sister, he would never have survived. She was such a great motivator that she could revive his zest to live a reasonable life.

Reflections
Early detection is much talked about and emphasized today. It is well-known that obesity can bring about many health complications. Unless a person takes early action, this is where life could go. Managing diabetes with medications, diet, and exercise can save a person if diabetes is detected early.

Monitoring all aspects of health thereafter is the only way to live well with the disease. Strictly following physician advice and keeping consistent with one's treatment is most important. Diabetes has no known cure. It can only be treated.

DETERMINATION MAKES HER WIN! – MARY SLONE

Mary Slone was discussing career options with friends one evening. When they turned to her to ask which career was of interest to her, she surprised them. "I want to be a pharmacist. It's a very good way to understand the quality of medicines, and you get to ensure that they are properly and lawfully made available." All her friends were impressed with her ambitious plans. The twenty-year-old was very aspiring and a very loving person, and she was universally loved.

One evening when getting ready for a family dinner, Mary noticed a butterfly-shaped rash on her cheeks. It kept bothering her that it was on her face and marring her looks.

Conscious of her appearance, she consulted a dermatologist, who diagnosed her with lupus, an autoimmune disease. She was prescribed medications including Plaquenil and Imuran to control her disease. But the disease flared up gradually, progressively affecting her blood and joints and leading to kidney failure.

She had just graduated from college and was admitted to the University's Pharmacy School. She made a very considered choice of peritoneal dialysis that would give her time to study and take control of her health. While others in her institute could focus on their studies and enjoy a carefree life, Mary had no time for any social life.

To be on a par with her classmates, Mary had to work very hard. She spent significant time on peritoneal dialysis and was regular with clinic visits so she could monitor her medical condition and have follow-up meetings with her kidney specialist. None of this got in the way of her achieving her goal.

"Congratulations, Pharmacist Mary! You conquered lupus!" Her physician welcomed her into the clinic with a huge smile. On his table was a cake. "We need to celebrate. You're one of my best patients. Many people leave school as if chronic kidney disease means the end of life. But, Mary, you never succumbed to any external pressures," he concluded. It was a happy hour with the doctor who always encouraged her with kind words. It was an emotional moment for Mary. But back home too there was a huge celebration.

Her heart swelled with happiness. Mary had become a pharmacist!

Through her life she faced unexpected trials, which sometimes left her depressed. But it was with great grit that she fought those moments, never letting hope for survival leave her side. Mary's deep faith, her family support, and the encouragement she received from her kidney specialist and nurses enabled her to meet new challenges courageously. All of them had participated in her success with joy.

Further treatments of immunosuppressant therapy and other relevant medications were given as required. Despite multiple blood pressure medications, Mary's blood pressure was uncontrollable. She was hospitalized after a massive stroke. She required assisted ventilation and stroke management in the ICU.

The worst after effect of the stroke was that she could no longer continue with her peritoneal dialysis. So after five years Mary moved on to hemodialysis. There she had to cope with a catabolic state, and management of severe electrolyte and fluid balance.

While in the ICU, Mary was treated by a group of physicians including a neurologist. Revival from coma seemed a remote possibility, but the family and her kidney specialist left no stone unturned. Unexpectedly she made recovery. After weeks of hospitalization in the ICU and two months in a rehabilitation center, her condition returned to normal.

On hemodialysis for about two years, Mary is stable and has no clinically detectable residual neurologic deficit. Soon she is expected to receive her license to practice. She is aware that dialysis is her lifeline, and she prefers peritoneal dialysis over hemodialysis, though she would rather live with anyone of them.. She is eagerly awaiting her chance for kidney transplantation.

Sheer determination helped Mary to manage lupus and complete the education she dreamed of. With chronic kidney disease, it has commonly been found that youth and young adults quit pursuing their education and leave lucrative jobs, many times encouraged by elder family members. Such actions arise out of a deep fear of loss of life, as managing the disease is very difficult. The value of finishing one's education and keeping a job that generates income has to be subtly promoted to patients and their family members. Everything rests on the patient's shoulders. Disease management is better when the person is emotionally positive and strives to overcome the disease and all limitations that supposedly accompany it.

A person with kidney disease needs emotional boosting, encouragement, and sufficient resources to deal with unexpected treatment costs. Mary was passionate about her career, so she made herself sufficiently secure to face the disease and medical costs. People around her were impressed. They were willing donors who supported her survival plans.

YOU CAN SET YOUR OWN BOUNDARIES
– JIMMY MCGRAW

Jimmy McGraw was a man with a happy disposition. He believed that life was to be lived fully, without any curb on his long hiking trips. The joy of the outdoors always excited him. Working as a civil engineer in a top-notch building construction company added scope for his travel. He did amazing work as an engineer and was quite a favorite among family and friends.

When Jimmy retired from work in 1973, his recreation time was extended beyond everybody's imaginations. Friends were amazed by his energy. As much as they tried, they failed to match his zest. He enjoyed a very fruitful life with a large family of five sons, five daughters, and many grandchildren and great-grandchildren. He traveled widely to forty-seven states within the United States, Mexico, and Canada by RV, making each trip a memorable and exciting experience.

It was toward the end of 2002 that he developed subtle symptoms suggestive of coronary artery disease. A coronary angiogram confirmed serious coronary disease. He underwent quadruple bypass. Unfortunately, his condition became complicated and morphed into a congestive heart failure. His kidneys quit working. He was referred to a kidney specialist for further evaluation.

"Jimmy, as much as I hate to say it, and although your physical condition has improved and you are feeing fit and strong, your kidneys are damaged. You will need to start dialysis very soon."

Jimmy decided against the kidney specialist's recommendation to start dialysis. Adopting persuasive and rational methods, the specialist convinced the ninety-year-old gentleman to try dialysis before making any long-term decision.

This strategy proved successful. After his first dialysis treatment, Jimmy felt more energetic. Gradually he adopted the schedule given by the doctor. As soon as his health improved, Jimmy used his boyish charm to convince the doctor to permit him a weekend break so he would travel in his RV.

In the RV, Jimmy resumed his regular escapades traveling around the country. He is active, walks short distances, and gets political news updates from the television. At ninety-six years of age, he has been on dialysis for more than five years.

Though Jimmy never liked dialysis, which he believes compromised his freedom, he never got depressed. And he is compliant with medications and diet to the satisfaction of his doctor.

A healthy mind maketh a healthy body. With kidney disease, not much health improvement can be achieved. But being happy through dialysis takes away the burden of the disease and reduces the patient's sorrow. Jimmy's escapades made living with dialysis far easier.

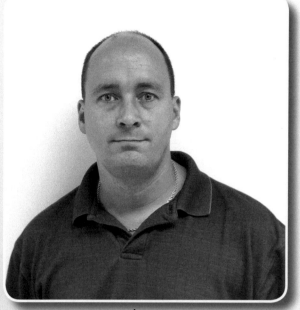

Eric Lee (Altruistic Donor)

A RARE HEAVENLY ENCOUNTER – ERIC LEE

Under a thick layer of bedcovers, Eric rolled restlessly. His face was distorted with stress. Beads of sweat broke out on his forehead, sending a strong early signal. In a few minutes he kicked his strong legs, struggling to break loose. As the agitation increased, he sat up, shaking compulsively, tossing aside the bedsheets. Mona stirred in bed, her eyes still heavy with sleep. She murmured, "What's up hon … ey?"

Eric's heavy breathing, escaping from his lips noisily, was enough for Mona to get out of bed, sleep lingering on her heavy eyelids. Eric's body was shaking violently.

Under the calming effect of her soft touch, Eric began gasping, slowly releasing his anguish. Mona poured out some water and extended the glass to her husband. A few sips of water seemed to help him calm a bit, but he spoke as if under the strain of a traumatic experience.

"It was a dream, so powerful, so real, unlike any I have had before."

"Tell me, Eric," she coaxed him, suppressing her own fears.

When Eric sat stunned, looking straight ahead, she continued her attempt to break through his silence, saying softly yet firmly, "Eric, all your life you dreamt such explosive dreams, sometimes of the past and sometimes of the future. So what's new?"

"She is dying, you know, and I need to help her soon," Eric said nervously, choking on his words.

"Eric, tell me exactly what happened!" Mona said in a firm tone, her eyes filled with concern, while she gently stroked him. She knew Eric too well to take this dream lightly.

"I saw a woman. Somehow I seemed to know her, as if we were friends. At first she looked fine. She appeared to be African American. That's what it seemed in there, in my dream." He looked at his wife to see if she believed him. She always did, but this dream was somehow different.

"Her husband was a Caucasian, with a distinctly 'funny' personality. She was very pleasant, but very quiet," Eric said reflectively.

"But something happened. Suddenly I could sense that the atmosphere had changed, but I didn't notice what had made that happen. Now, it was no longer friendly. It was sad and depressing all around. There was a visible change. I looked at my friend and saw her getting hooked up to a machine, with a connection on her arm. Tubes leading from the machine stuck here." He pointed to his right arm below the elbow, looking at the place strangely as if needles were stuck there.

"When I looked up, I observed the change on her face. She looked very unhappy now. Eventually I was no longer able to speak with her."

He paused. Then as if remembering the event and linking it to the woman's sadness, he said, "I saw her going for treatments several times. Plenty of treatment. I couldn't understand what was wrong with her.

"And then. I turned my head and saw myself lying in a pale blue hospital gown on a sterile metallic operating table. The doctors were performing a surgery of some kind. I was lying still and there were doctors and nurses around. Then I saw vividly an incision on my lower left side, a long cut just below my waistline.

"And within minutes I saw my friend receiving what they took from me." Eric looked peculiarly at his wife; whether he was puzzled or scared, one couldn't gather from Eric's expression. "What could it be?" he asked into space, hoping someone would give him a clue.

Mona had been watching him closely throughout the entire time he spoke. She quickly prompted, "You need to write it down now. In the morning you can speak to a doctor to find out what that procedure was that you saw in your dream."

After some silence, Eric resumed talking. "I have recorded all my past dreams, when they were still fresh, so they are accurate. But this one … I hope that, if it were possible to transfer what I have seen into visual transcripts that could be reproduced for display on a screen, it will be seen in true dimension. It was so real—just very scary!" He shook his shoulders as if to shoo the dream away.

"Tell me more, Eric," his wife goaded, adding pressure by gripping his hand tighter.

"I never dwell on them too much, but I've always believed that many of my dreams have some link with my life in some way."

"I know," she said vaguely, as her mind recalled many such past dreams.

Now, fully aroused, Eric did just what his wife had suggested. The next few days Eric spent in gathering information. He found out that what he'd dreamt about was a laparoscopic surgery for a kidney transplant, which was minimally invasive and yielded a quick recovery. It was less painful than scalpel surgery too!

He read about kidney disease, how patients suffer because of insufficient kidney function, restrictive diet, and the morbidity of the disease.

Eric went into frenzy, digging deeper. He needed more relevant information. What did kidney patients need most? In the process he found out that Federal Law prohibited financial compensation for kidney donation. Contributions came by way of people giving of their time to conduct fund-raising events, which Eric had heard of before. The most significant act was to give a part of oneself unselfishly to bring about a dramatic change in a kidney patient's life. The trials experienced during dialysis, the long wait for the allotment of a kidney, and ultimately the truth stood naked before him.

He should donate his kidney to someone who was facing danger of extinction.

Eric discussed the organ donation with Mona and his two teenage daughters, in what was a heartrending, overwhelming conversation. His earnestness while explaining the unique opportunity to help someone, his sharing risk factors of the surgery and recovery times, and his concluding that it was his heart's call won him unilateral support for such an altruistic cause. It was his parents' worry that left Eric uncomfortable. Though he understood their concerns, he knew there was no way he would change his mind.

During the process of discussion, his determination reached its peak.

Active search for a "worthy" patient began. He watched videos of people looking for a kidney donor. Eric was amazed at the simple process. He'd never known anyone personally with kidney disease, so now reading about people who had it left him horrified that large numbers of these people lived in desperation. Mona and Eric found it extremely difficult to nail down a patient. Instead of finding the woman he had dreamed about, Eric left it to God to find the right candidate.

One morning he walked into Yale New Haven Hospital's transplant unit, offering to be a living donor. He expressed his sense of urgency to get the surgery done. Eric did not want any untoward incident to spoil this mission. With great speed, a coordinator was assigned to Eric and the process began.

The first piece of information, namely, that his blood group was O, meant that his kidney could go to patients in any blood group, but if a person had type O blood, then he would be in desperate need, as people in the O blood group can only receive from another person with type O. Eric's family understood the full implications that a person with type O blood must wait a long time for a kidney.

In the months ahead, Eric played enthusiastically the game of donor evaluation. He underwent more tests, scans, interviews (psychiatric and psychological), and physical examinations.

All this time, some ninety miles away from Connecticut, in Cheshire, Lisa was on a tight schedule with thrice-a-week dialysis. With great effort, every alternate weekday she dragged herself to the clinic.

Being on dialysis for seven long years was taking its toll. Her energy levels were gradually seeing a drop. But being very sensible, she knew that continuing with dialysis was only way she would survive.

One evening she returned home after a session and collapsed on the couch. Her husband Al was shocked to see her in such a state. He did everything he could make her comfortable. But seeing her on slumped on the couch had him worried—extremely worried.

That night as she lay in bed, every ounce of energy spent, she sent out a plea: "Lord, please find me a donor. This is how much I can manage to do."

The next morning, Lisa was clearing the breakfast table. Then she had a second cup of black coffee. Her mind was clouded with many thoughts. Loud ringing from the telephone broke through her reverie.

The caller said, "Hey there. I am Susan Richard calling from the Yale New Haven Hospital. I need to speak to Lisa, please."

"Yes, this is Lisa."

"Hey, Lisa, how are you doing? We have some good news for you. We have found a matching donor for you. Congratulations. Can you come over tomorrow at 11:00 a.m. to meet with the transplant team?"

With as much energy as she could gather, Lisa said, "Yes, I will." Somewhere inside, she felt her heart was ready to burst, while she felt a certain tremor and nervousness deep within..

She fiddled with the phone and called Al.

"I got it, Al. It's come. Hospital called. Tomorrow at 11:00 a.m. we need to meet."

In a few days, in early August, Eric got a message: "We have found a recipient with a perfect match. The surgery date is fixed for August 10."

Eric learned it was a woman from Connecticut who'd been on dialysis for seven years.

It was a Tuesday morning. In spite of a bright sun smiling down, Eric was shivering with nervousness, but he was also excited.

As he finished the paperwork at the registration office, Eric, turning, saw a man wheeling a woman in a wheelchair. Struck by her familiarity, Eric said softly, "That's her." Mona turned, a bit too late. All she saw was a receding wheelchair going in the opposite direction.

In the recovery room Eric was informed that the surgery was successful.

Finally when he broke through the effects of anesthesia, Eric found himself in a room with happily smiling faces bending over him. Seeing his parents, he knew that in spite of their initial hesitation, their faith in him had remained intact.

In a few days, Eric returned to normal life. He had an extraordinary feeling of peace for having given a body part to change someone's way of life. He experienced some unusual moments of elation, almost feeling he was a soldier returning home from war.

In early December a letter arrived in his mailbox. Eric was completely taken aback. It was from Lisa. What she wrote was so soothing. Unexpectedly, tears of joy and excitement began to flow. She wanted to meet him.

Under the rules for kidney donation, he had agreed not to seek out his kidney recipient. But this was a happy surprise.

Closer to Christmas, Eric was invited by Lisa to her Christmas party. She called it a surprise, as she would not reveal the identity of the special party guest.

The evening of the party, Eric found himself standing outside the main door, a bundle of nerves, excited. It took a moment and a deep breath for him to knock on the heavy wood door.

As the door opened, Eric saw standing on the threshold the woman from his dream. Yes, it was her; the woman who had entered his dream, the very same person. The pieces of the puzzle fit perfectly. It had been her all throughout, at the hospital in the wheelchair and in the adjacent operating room waiting for his kidney.

His eyes brimmed with tears. This was something beyond his capacity to understand and digest. He marveled at it. The union was a very emotional experience for both of them. As they embraced, a new relationship formed, one of love. Lisa became part of Eric's extended family.

But now, Eric saw his role emerging as an advocate for organ donation. In the past few months, many aspects of the disease had come into his consciousness that he could not drive away. He was on the warpath to spread word of the value of kidney donation.

As Eric came closer to Lisa, he learned that Al had offered to donate his kidney, but because of a blood mismatch, the offer was turned down. Eric impressed upon Al that he should choose to donate to another patient in need.

Sometimes when Eric recalls his dream, his chest swells with pride. He feels proud that things fell into place, that he had managed to reenact the story as it unveiled itself in his dream.

All he did was made a choice. It changed someone's life forever.

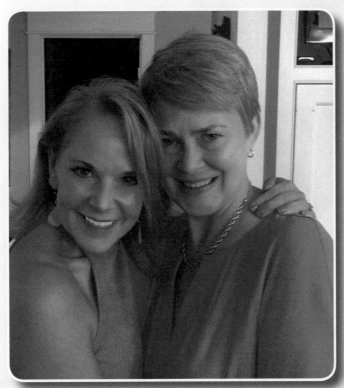

Left: Amy Otto (Altruistic Donor)
Right: Rebecca Springer (Transplantee)

STRIKING THE RIGHT CHORD – AMY AND BECKY

Amy Otto was busy scheduling official meetings for April.

Suddenly she stopped. "Oh! Becky's birthday is in April. How could I forget it?" She bit her lower lip, reprimanding herself. She scribbled on her planner, "Becky's birthday—gift to be ordered," and sat thinking of her fairly new friend, who inspired her in more ways than one.

As she drove home from work, she passed her favorite spa. In a flash, a fleeting thought turned into an interesting idea. Taking the service road, she maneuvered into an empty parking space. Once inside the aromatic spa, she checked the packages they offered. Amy chose one she had used before. She walked to the front desk, ready to place the order. The manager at the desk smiled at Amy warmly. "Hey. How are you today?"

Amy smiled and responded, "Hey. Nice to see you. I was wondering if you could spare a few moments. I want to buy a gift for a very dear friend, Becky Springer. I will fill out the form, but I need to speak to you and discuss some important aspects."

Taking her aside, Amy explained Becky's situation. From the change in expression on the manager's face, Amy could see her concern. The manager quickly assured Amy. "Our customers find our personalized treatment awesome, as we make it an ultimate joy for them. Your friend will be made completely at ease. She will enjoy it. I am very sure about that," she said with confidence, her freshly trimmed bob bouncing.

Amy walked out overjoyed. *What a perfect gift!*

Good. Becky needs to be pampered! She will simply love being in such a soothing aromatic atmosphere. The fragrances …hmm, she thought, completely convinced that no other gift would be better.

Amy was excited. "That's how I felt, wonderfully spoiled and pampered when Chuck surprised me with a spa gift last year." She grinned, remembering her own exhilarating experience, including the glow on her face when she walked into the restaurant for a romantic dinner later that evening. "Life is just a few moments of joy," she mused.

As she drove home, she recalled their first meeting, how the friendship had developed. A book club of her mom's in an Atlanta suburb drew a group of women together monthly to discuss a book, enjoy wine, and engage in some good conversation. Amy had been a part of the book club for about a year when they welcomed a new member, Becky.

Becky, gushing with life, was smart and funny. She participated actively in the discussions, and her exuberance was infectious. It was easy for Amy to break the ice with her. Soon they became good friends, sharing many common things. Their friendship was simply pure and unassuming, with no strings attached. Amy admired Becky's capabilities and was astounded by her joy for life. Her interest in Becky was so heightened that she had taken every opportunity to get to know her better. She looked into the car mirror and smiled. Now their early days of friendship seemed so long ago.

That evening as Amy was setting the dinner table, Chuck noticed her looking exceptionally happy. He raised his brows expectantly. Bubbling with eagerness, she spoke of what she had done.

"Ah, so you're planning Becky Springer's surprise birthday gift," Andi chipped in from behind, winking at her brother while teasing her mom. Between gurgles of laughter, they recalled an earlier surprise gift that had gone totally wrong. The dinner became a hilarious affair with many anecdotes of surprise parties and gifts.

But after dinner, and on a serious note, Amy narrated some major life-changing events in Becky's life. Their stomachs full, the family gave half an ear until the story reached its finale.

"It happened just after Valentine's Day in 2008. Becky felt a chill. She wore a cardigan when city temperatures were normal. That evening while trying to dial the phone, she realized her fingers had grown stiff; they simply would not flex. Alarmed, Paul had rushed her to the ER. She was admitted into the hospital for a checkup.

"The next morning when Becky regained consciousness, a shattered Paul was trying to explain why she was in the hospital. Up to that time, Becky was unaware that her hands and feet were no longer there! They'd been amputated in an emergency surgery as the best resort under the circumstances. Can you predict her reaction?"

Amy stole a glance around the table. Now she saw her family members moving uneasily in their seats as if they were roused. It's not that Amy anticipated any reaction other than surprise. Her eyes sparkled with pride as she continued pouring out the heart-wrenching story, her voice modulated to inspire her family.

"Unexpectedly Becky acted differently. She received the news calmly, unquestioningly. No wailing, no anger—none of the usual explosive behavior. Isn't that amazing! An anxious doctor explained to her the diagnosis, saying that Becky was a victim of *Haemophilus influenzae* type B, known as Hib.

"The terrible infection first attacked her organs. Her kidneys were first to shut down. It led to septicemia, a serious, life-threatening condition caused by bacteria in the blood. A stroke had paralyzed her. To prevent further onslaughts by the infection, her hands and feet had been sacrificed.

"After six weeks at the Rehabilitation Institute of Chicago, Becky regained her strength. It began with her being on twenty-four-hour dialysis, now reduced to thrice a week."

Amy sipped some water to calm her nerves. Then she concluded, "Back in Atlanta, she continues with dialysis."

The family was stunned into silence. Becky's story was so startling, unreal. It was impossible to listen to, understand, and digest it and then think normally.

Chuck remarked, "It amazes me how Becky faced it with such nonchalance. One would feel the carpet had been pulled out from beneath their feet."

After a few minutes he added more, as if he were making an assessment. "Such an upheaval would destroy the fabric of any family, as the hands that held the family together were Becky's, and now they are gone! That's women's power, to stand firmly rooted to preserve their families during adversity. If Becky had buckled, her family would be down in the sands."

All in the room felt their hearts miss a beat as they searched their souls. They were left with deep pools of emotion, call it pride, or sympathy, or awe, upon seeing someone larger than life. Becky's brave front left them speechless. They were humbled by her fight to survive and were overcome by respect. In a sudden flash they understood Amy's unquestionable attachment to her new friend. No wonder, given the exceptional quality of their mother's friendship and what had kindled it.

April arrived, and along with it came Becky's birthday. Amy had made subtle references to Becky about a surprise outing followed by lunch. Everything was planned. Both women longed for their hour-long chat over a leisurely lunch.

Amy was right in anticipating Becky's joy upon discovering the special treat that awaited her at the spa. It was all very exciting. Soon some great surprises unfolded that caught Amy off guard. It started with the gown being handed over for her to change into. Becky whispered to Amy, "Can you please come with me?"

As they moved to the changing room, Amy realized that Becky would need some help. Gradually, to prepare for the session, Becky had to remove the prosthetics, before she could finally get upon the table. Amy was struck by the small structure of the table. She smiled, willing herself to remain composed.

The attendant came in, dimmed the lights, and said to her prospect enthusiastically, "Becky, let's get you completely relaxed. We'll begin with a hand massage."

"I have no hands!" Becky stated simply, unflinching.

"Oh my, then let's start with your legs," the aesthetician said, changing course.

"I don't have feet!"

Suddenly being made aware that the person on her table had no movable limbs, the attendant burst into tears, rushing out in utter shock. The manager hadn't explained Becky's case to her.

Amy patted Becky's arm and then followed the woman into the lobby. Seeing the woman's body shaking with emotion, Amy spoke soothingly. "It's okay, you know. No problem. But you must calm yourself. Try to forget this incident and start afresh. It's her birthday, so we must make it super special. Give her a facial that she will enjoy. This is her first date at a spa after her accident—and she simply loves to be pampered."

With prompting from Amy, the attendant went back and brightened the room with her smile, asking for Becky's preference of fragrance, tucking a towel here, raising the bed, and making Becky comfortable.

Leaving the duo, Amy slipped out.

Once in the confines of the private space of her car, she started the ignition. She couldn't believe how small Becky appeared without her prosthetic legs. How challenged must Becky feel every day of her life! By now Amy's body was shaking; she was sobbing at her own inadequacy and not being to handle her emotions. Warm tears rolled down her checks in torrents, inconsolable pain wracking her mind and body. Crying to quell her thumping heart, Amy was moaning for her friend's loss, so many years later, in which time Becky had conquered many fears and lived through dark phases when many personal aspirations had crashed and burned.

Amy was very confused. What to think? What to do? She shifted uncomfortably in the car seat, trying to get her thoughts clear, all the while hugging her body to shield it against an unknown fear.

Poor Becky. No, I can't use that word for her. But, God, how is she able to handle so much? We are both very similar, like mother and daughter or like sisters. But she has so many challenges to handle!

In a flash, some bits of conversation between them came back:

"I found it most difficult to learn to walk again. But using the prosthetic hands was simply impossible."

The agony raised Amy's heartbeat. Becky occupied her thoughts. How many problems her friend suffered in her everyday life.

As she sat huddled behind the wheel, Amy made a decision. She would help her friend in every way she could. Suddenly she felt in control. She walked back to the spa in a happy frame of mind. Over lunch with Becky, she steered the conversation.

Becky mentioned an article she had recently read about a new type of hand transplant that could restore for a recipient complete control over movement of their fingers. "If I just had a right hand, life would be considerably easier." Becky sighed.

"But it's a kidney transplant that I desperately need. They've had me on the national list since 2009, and as yet no matching donor has been found. I am a difficult match because of the trauma my body has undergone," Becky said, unflustered by the way the conversation was going.

After lunch they did some clothes shopping. Becky had weight issues. On weekends she gained ten to fifteen pounds because of the long gap between dialysis sessions. So with Amy's help, Becky tried on clothes and bought some loose dresses.

Throughout the entire time they shopped, events of the day and pieces of conversation played on Amy's mind. The next day she called Piedmont Hospital, where Becky was registered, and made an appointment with the nephrologist.

It was a few days later, when Becky and her nurse were readying for dialysis, when Paul came downstairs hesitantly. For convenience and better quality of life, Becky had changed to peritoneal dialysis. The machine was installed in the basement. "Becky, the hospital called. They have a willing live donor. Your blood needs to be drawn for a tissue match. Identity of the prospect is undisclosed. So we may have a surprise!" His eyes were shining brightly. He even winked at her.

Becky felt a knot forming in her stomach. But as always, her mind ruled over heart, enough for her to recognize it was pointless to raise her expectations. She would wait for positive signs. Her thoughts hovered around her life and family, especially her three wonderful daughters, Ashley, Mary Catherine, and Gretchen.

How devastated they were when I returned without my limbs. But they quickly assumed additional responsibilities. Ashley took her role as eldest very seriously, but Mary and Gretch were also helpful. God has given me such valuable gems. Oh well. We managed, thanks to Paul, who was most burdened!

Her eyes were moist, and her lips spread into a smile.

Five years have flown by. Now Ashley is grown into a young lady, Mary is in her teens, and Gretch is still almost a kid. Hmm!

Heaving a big sigh, she settled down to the reality of being dialyzed. A few hours later she would be planning the family meal.

Amy was busy with an important meeting when the call came. She took her call and was spellbound to hear that she was found to be a perfect match. But the hospital representative added that it was highly improbable to have such a perfect match; the test could be wrong. They were scheduling a repeat test soon.

At some point in time Becky became privy to the highly confidential information that it was Amy who had tested and that, most wonderfully, her tissue, on all six parameters, was a spot-on match with Becky's.

But Amy and Becky faced many trying moments of uncertainty. The doctors were not satisfied that a 100 percent match was possible. Somehow repeated tests revealed the same results. Amy had to follow the protocol process for kidney transplant evaluation. She was occupied with the variety of scans, x-rays, ultrasounds, and other tests.

Finally Amy was able to donate the kidney on June 3, 2011.

As Becky's new kidney kicked in, urine forming, her skin changed color from ash, to pale yellow, to bright pink. It had a healthy glow. Happiness spread around, as this dramatic change was noticeable.

Some months later, Becky reflected on how although personally life had changed for her with the kidney transplant, Ashley, Mary Catherine, and Gretchen had not shown any great enthusiasm. It struck her that the kidney helped her lead a normal life as far as diet, passing urine normally, and importantly not having to undergo dialysis went, but her girls did not see it bring any change to their lives. If Becky could get back her hands and legs, that would be a significant change and bring smiles to their faces.

Yes, she should work toward that.

It was the last week of March 2014. Becky reached out to pick up her new cell phone that had beeped loud.

"Hey, Becky," said the warm and friendly voice, one that Becky could recognize even in her sleep.

"Oh … Hey, Amy. What's up?"

She continued excitedly, "Remember the patch with orchids that I am growing? So, they look amazing! … You must come by. I am watering them as I speak with you."

A few minutes later they spoke of other things, about the family, and then Becky could finally say what mattered most to her. "Amy, every day I think of it. I want to say it now. God sent you to me. We met for a purpose. You came into my life to be the kidney donor who was such a perfect match.

"I have no other explanation for our friendship, Amy. Thank you so much for being there for me!"

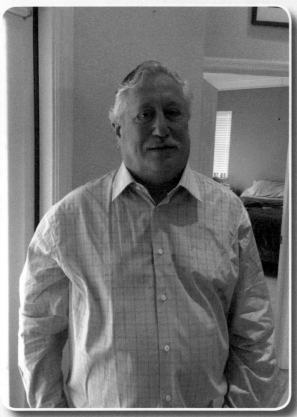
Mark Rosen (Maintenance Treatment)

HIDE-AND-SEEK WITH CREATININE – MARK ROSEN

"What does a man do when suddenly a stranger knocks at the door?" said Mark, smiling at his friend. "'I'm the cancer in your right kidney' is what the stranger said," he said nonchalantly.

The friend was dumbstruck at first. "What happened, Mark?" he asked with disbelief.

Mark said, "'Shoo, go away!' I barked. I was quickly admitted to the hospital. After going through detailed discussions, the right kidney was surgically removed."

Of course Mark knew what it meant to have an organ removed, but the emotional waves that kept him ravaged were something he had to deal with. His wife Patty proved to be his greatest supporter. She bravely held his hand through the ordeal, making it a less harsh reality.

The year 2010 went flying by. Mark opened a fresh diary in January 2011, summoning his strength and self-motivation to move on.

"I'm not letting cancer determine my life. It can't kill my seafarer's spirit, or prevent me from sailing and fishing in Alaska! My love for life in the blue waters—what peace it gives me!"

But Mark grew very sincere about maintaining his health. On the doctor's advice, he did a battery of tests, wonderingly, yet hoping that it was the last of his hospital visits.

Seeing his lab reports, Mark noticed higher levels for creatinine. So the meeting with the nephrologist was not going to be fun. Shaking his head, the nephrologist confirmed that Mark was having an issue with his kidney; he was at stage 4 of kidney disease.
Mark felt as if the sword of Damocles was now hanging just above his head, waiting to axe him at any time. It frightened him to his wits' end. Every three months he needed to go and get his tests done. If the kidney function fell below 15 percent, the doctor said he would need dialysis.

Patty was equally disturbed. It was important to understand what triggered creatinine. Proactively, she researched how to postpone dialysis.

Both Mark and Patty were absolutely clear: Mark should be spared from having to undergo dialysis by maintaining the kidney's function as presented by this test.

Patty was spot-on when she discovered that the key driver of the disease was diet. If they could nail down the best diet to manage creatinine, they would be saved from great hardships. Armed with this revelation, they approached the nephrologist seeking a recommendation for a good renal dietician.

It took a few weeks for the doctor to direct them to a renal dietician. For some reason the dietician shared very limited information. It gave the couple little confidence to meet the challenge of a life-threatening disease.

"This is so confusing. We are left with nothing but fear! Such peripheral information for this disease," Mark spoke out, as soon as he could come out of his state of shock. "Will I be able to lead a safe life without dialysis?"

Then he began exploratory work, even when other disturbing thoughts chased his mind.

Suddenly a conversation with a friend gave the couple a clue and a new direction. At first it was difficult to comprehend, but research helped.

And then voilá! Or you could say it was an 'Eureka moment'.

Mark decided to start a Facebook page. It began as a learning process, gaining information about kidney disease and a renal diet. Slowly people at various stages of kidney disease joined. They would ask questions, to which Mark had quick replies. It was a learning and sharing group. Many members shared some great information they had gathered during their rough ride through unknown territory.

Gradually the Facebook group grew larger and provided more focused information. Discussions happened. The group grew to about eleven hundred members from the world over. Everyone was there to help and support each other.

As the group grew, Mark was also making many decisions about his diet and health. From the lab reports, he felt he understood the renal diet and also learned a lot about the disease. When trying to explain his diet, Mark would say he kept mostly the same diet but would cheat sometimes. But within a short time he would bounce back onto the proven track. Fortunately it helped him.

His diet was simply tailored to match his lab results. He had to keep all parameters within acceptable levels.

If you were to flip through Mark's diary, the abstract would keep you mesmerized. Mark recorded his plans, his thought process, and how through simple tweaking of diet he achieved some good results. Following is a sample from Mark's diary.

Date, eGFR*, and creatinine	Action plan / observations
January 2011 – 19%	
August 2011 – 19% to 32%	Credit: Diet and exercise. Walking three to seven miles a day. I tell my teammates, "This does take work, but we have to look at what we want in life! For me, it's to be able to live—to fish, hunt, or just play with the grandchildren. I want a productive life. So I continue the fight for health. We can do this together and learn from each other. Just one more thing: I am very proactive with my health. I have my blood work done each month, so I know how I am doing. I was also told I have multiple myeloma and that turned out to be okay and then I was told I have lupus, and that too is not a problem for me."
September 23, 2012 – eGFR down to 21% from 27%	I do not know what I am doing to make this happen. Still eating and exercising. Just more stress and depression set in, but now it seems to be gone.
December 15, 2012 – eGFR 31.8%; creatinine 2.1	Blood pressure went up; now it is normal.
January 8, 2013	Tomorrow I have appointments with a urologist, an oncologist, and a nephrologist. Feeling a little nervous.
January 9, 2013 – eGFR 30%; creatinine 2.2	
April 2013 – eGFR down to 26%	

May 2013 – eGFR 34%	Only change—cut out chicken and turkey from my diet. Now eating only fish.
June 2013 – eGFR 32%; creatinine 2.0	Dietary changes made. Moved to mostly veggie diet. Fish three times a week. Tough, but I felt it would be worth the effort.
August 2013	New nephrologist wants blood work every three months. Feels good to be in stage 3. Not stressing as before. Have let go of my past; dealing with each moment as it comes. I know for me it is important to stay hydrated, to eat a healthy renal diet, and to exercise daily. But keeping stress down for me is a top priority.
December 30, 2013 – eGFR of 32%	Will be changing my diet again to see if these changes help improve my numbers!
January 10, 2014 – eGFR 25%	Doctor testing me for everything—scans, blood tests—trying to figure out what is going on. MRI and seeing oncologist in two weeks. The fun begins again …
February 26, 2014 – eGFR was 28%	Try to get back to 30%. Low white blood cells. Is my multiple myeloma still active?
May 2, 2014 – eGFR down from 34% to 25%	On May 7, twenty-four-hour urine test and blood work. I hope to see improvements.
May 17, 2014 – eGFR is back to the 30% range	Bad news: likely liver problem. Doctor has ordered another lab test for next week.
June 26, 2014 – eGFR back up to 30%	Got a call from my doctor. My liver function is normal. Stress, stress, and then back to normal.
July 1, 2014	Given up Facebook. I just don't feel I have the ability to help anyone anymore. The stress of the groups daily is upsetting me. I worry about my inability to help heal all. Not even able to heal myself. Children with kidney disease is hard for me. Boy, I only wish I had a kidney give to them all.
July 15, 2014 – eGFR is 39%	*Wow!* Today's results, what a joy!
September 9, 2014 – eGFR 40%; creatinine 1.72	Thanks to all of you for your help.

October 20, 2014 – eGFR 41%; creatinine 1.6	Doing better than last month. Wow, this is amazing. So happy.
November 25, 2014 – eGFR went from 41% down to 38%	Okay, what happened? I was dehydrated. Will work hard on hydration. Am I worried? No, not at all. This is kidney disease; it will have many ups and downs. It can do me much more harm if I start to obsess about all of this. So T-Day is coming—holiday time, family time. Just enjoy your time. —Mark Rosen
February 15, 2015	Changed my diet—from a raw diet back to cooked. Having diarrhea. Not good. So I will see if I can improve with the change. I will be having blood tests on the eighteenth, and then next week I have an appointment with the nephrologist. Will update after doctor appointment.
February 24, 2015 – eGFR 41%; creatinine is 1.68	Labs keep improving, and again I feel it is hydration, diet and exercise, and keeping my stress low.
April 2, 2015 – eGFR is 41% (no change); creatinine 1.68—stage 3	Working to reach stage 2. Looking into what adjustments I can make to diet and exercise. Is this where it stops? Is this the best it gets for me? Can I reach this new goal of stage 2?
August 12, 2015 – eGFR went from 37% to 40% this time	This is proof to keep stress low in my life. Stress messes up my mind and body. Great improvement; very happy. All other doctor appointments went pretty well. Need to get more tests for liver. Thing here is that kidney function is improving again.
October 26, 2015 – eGFR 40%	Got home from oncologist. All labs very good. Liver is better and cancer number is better. I feel good today, thankful for my diet and how I keep improving.

November 23, 2015 – two weeks before, eGFR of 40%, and now 33%	Big movement ... why? Guessing it is the king crab eaten in between blood tests, which I felt gave me the gout. Am I right? But it is a good educated guess. Gout adds stress to the body. Anyway, will have to pull up my big-boy pants and make some major adjustments to diet! Maybe just have to practice more ways to get rid of the stress I give myself.
June 2016 – eGFR 36%	Doctor appointment today. Wow, it is a progressive disease. eGFR 36%. Not feeling good about this. Going up to four bicarbonate of soda a day now—650 mg. Will post more later. This is just the start ...
June 2017 – all steady, but pain in calf muscles	Manganese level is down. Need to improve it.

* estimated glomerular filtration rate

People like Mark Rosen seem to have a single thought process: *Keep kidney function tied down to the same spot.* But it was the toughest challenge for him. He tried to beat it down. It was managed for six years. And with tweaking his diet he continued to fight it down.

The road for kidney patients is a tough one. But lesser-traveled roads will keep you inspired and keep you wanting more.

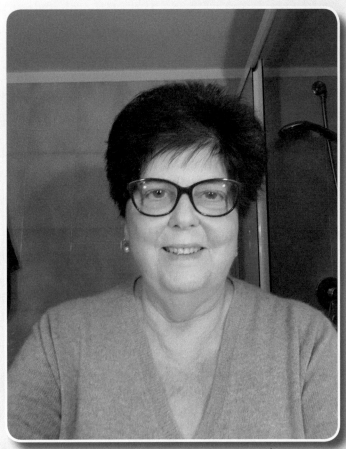

Magda Bonacina (Preemptive Transplantee)

WAR WAGING WITHIN – MAGDA BONACINA, ITALY

Six-year-old Magda pulled her scarf tight, closer around her neck, as if guarding something. *Mama asked me to keep the cold morning air away!* she thought as she looked at the gray, fog-laden sky, which was making the road to her school less visible. Milan was always known to be a cold town with thick curtains of fog.

The chat and laughter around her drew her attention. She quickened her steps to walk with the girls. As her eyes moved from her shoes upward, she noticed that none of them wore pants. She was wearing what in modern times are called a panty hose, which were unheard of in those times in Italy as part of women's clothing.

But Mama says I should protect myself against the cold. I love school. I love walking with those girls, love their laughter and chatter … Why worry about my clothes being different? I must not fall ill. I hate to stay at home on school days.

She shrugged away all such random thoughts. "It doesn't matter!"

When her mother encouraged her to eat meat, saying, "You will keep warm and build resistance against cold and cough," Magda would look into the earnest eyes of her parents, Alma and Luciano, and force herself to eat as much as possible. Being frail, she was susceptible to colds. She was fed mostly on meat, in addition to good nutritious soups. Herbal teas were given to her when she was ill. Much effort was made to keep her well.

What was wrong with Magda? Was it the polluted environment from the period of the Second World War and after, in Milan?

The Second World War was perhaps the most poignant period in world history. This war, about soldiers, conspiracy, and calamities, also marked the birth of nuclear warfare, signifying a mysterious future. Living with terror in their hearts and with stories of violence inscribed in their minds left the people cold. Long drawn-out periods of warfare and the massive loss of life created deep wedges in people's hearts, wiping out love for their fellow humans.

During the war, families living near Milan's military camp battled with many problems. German forces had taken over Milan and converted the rubber and car engine factories into war weapon manufacturing units. Thick toxic smog turned blue skies to gray and also gave many civilians respiratory diseases. Intermittent coughing came to be recognized as tuberculosis, for which treatments were unheard of during that period.

Magda was a two-month-old baby when she contracted a whooping cough. Her parents were anxious and were in fear that it would be tuberculosis. But it turned out to be allergic asthma.

Luciano worked in a factory, and later he started writing for sports magazine, while Alma became a writer of history books for kids. They were both well-read and worldly-wise, so they did their own research.

In those days when bronchodilator sprays had not yet been invented, it was very tough to manage Magda's health. Alma wondered if Magda's asthma was a food-related allergy. In 1955 little was known of allergies and psychosomatic diseases. However, Alma's persistence helped her find an allergologist whose prescription of a steroid that could cure Magda's asthma seemed too drastic a treatment and risky. Alma quickly turned down that option for fear of its leading to an irreversible condition.

Taking the doctor's other suggestion seriously, Alma took Magda to a sea town where the weather was reasonable. Magda recuperated and went back to school a year later.

Waging a war with an invisible enemy was tough, but Alma trudged on. Suddenly it dawned on her. *Am I being obsessed about Magda's health? Should I spend time like a mother with a daughter, or only think of her asthma? I always wonder what to do next!*

Soul-searching confirmed the bitter truth. Determined as she was, Alma changed her attitude before it became a malady. Suddenly shaking her head, she decided, *Magda should become independent!*

Magda was sent to spend her vacation with relatives and friends.

Hesitant at first, Magda began enjoying outings with friends after a while. She learned how to manage her life. It was a new experience being in the company of young cousins and friends. They did many wonderful things together. An occasional cough was well managed by her. During her time away from home, she observed how elders around were carefree. With some guilt, she realized that her parents were very concerned about her health.

A period of learning began: managing health, being aware of what happened around her, and seeing people enjoy life, laughing, dancing, and eating anything at all.

They are lucky. They have no health worries! she thought, shrugging her shoulders indifferently.

And then Magda met Paolo during one of her mountain vacations. Their friendship grew deep and long lasting. In her final year of schooling, she contracted hepatitis A. Some fish she had consumed was the cause of the infection. Magda spent a year at home recovering. All that time she was aware that Paolo, studying to be a lawyer, was marching ahead. Guilt and determination were triggered, so Magda worked hard to complete her education. She consciously put her health on the back burner.

After graduation, she looked back at the rough road she had traversed, through thick fog of toxic air, all of which she had survived. All that seemed well worth it. Magda realized with an inward pride that in spite of her frequent tussles with asthma, she had made it!

Paolo was her man. They were married when she was twenty-two years old, and lived in Genova, on the Mediterranean coast. Paolo was kept busy in the court as a lawyer, while Magda began teaching at a high school. Her subjects were Italian literature, history, the ancient Latin language. She was also a part-time researcher at Genova University working on medieval Latin manuscripts.

Because it was discovered that Magda's father-in-law had a genetic disease, Paolo and Magda chose to adopt a child. Bringing up Michele, doing schoolwork, and attending to family responsibilities kept Magda busy. But her life's course changed in her thirty-eighth year. Suddenly old nightmares broke through their cage, threatening her peace and happiness. She came face-to-face with life's most harrowing moments.

It was a simple fever, with flulike symptoms. But when she found blood in her urine, she felt the ground beneath her feet give way.

Is this a sign of cancer? was her first thought.

It was only a single episode, but it was enough to freak her out completely. Even as this bizarre thought entered her mind, her mother's early training prodded her to unleash her weapon. She should find out more. At first the information was overwhelming, but gradually, when she realized she did not have cancer, she became more relaxed.

Blood in the urine is known as "gross hematuria." Magda met doctors and medical experts who were unable to give her any definite prognosis (even if they suspected it to be IgA nephropathy). It took nearly six years of searching to arrive at any conclusion. In 1990 a biopsy confirmed that Magda had Berger's disease, a type of IgA (an autoimmune disease).

A few years later, over afternoon tea, Paolo and Magda casually started a discussion that revolved around her IgA research.

Magda explained in a troubled voice, "Ninety percent of patients get diagnosed only after a casual episode of gross hematuria, because IgA is a silent disease. For some people it may take years for any symptom to surface. Another interesting part of IgA is that it could grow fast into a full-blown disease in some, whereas in others it is less aggressive, which means slow progression of the disease."

Paolo was amazed by the detailed information and knowledge that Magda had acquired. Looking into her clear, earnest eyes, he said encouragingly, "It means you have done so much work. Can you imagine what this information will mean to many people who don't understand the disease?"

"I know. I was lucky. And yes, I must share it with people." From the twinkle in her eye he could see he had ignited a purpose. He squeezed her hand, encouraging her to go all out spreading her knowledge.

Magda started with writing a blog. She became a member of IgA groups in Europe and the USA and participated in conferences. She became an advocate for people with IgA and became a group administrator on Facebook. Gradually, after having started out small, doing side work, Magda became a full-fledged campaigner for spreading awareness of the disease. As her role grew, she continuously learned more about IgA. Some important points about IgA are as follows:

- It is a genetic autoimmune mediated disorder that affects the kidneys, when the genetic anomalies are triggered by some external factor (such as infection, vaccines, or a virus).
- It is genetic but not directly hereditary. It can run in families (especially in Asian families).
- Usually it manifests after an episode of respiratory infection, cough, and cold. Apart from cola-colored urine, other symptoms are back pain below the ribs, protein in the urine, swelling in the hands and feet, and sometimes digestive issues.
- IgA's antibodies are generated in the mucus of the respiratory tract and in intestinal mucus.
- IgA's antibodies get deposited into the glomeruli gradually, but it impacts kidney function at a slow rate. In most cases it is not aggressive and there is no definitive treatment.

Magda's own reaction to her episode of hematuria and what she gathered in her research made her draw some definite conclusions, as follows:

- Seeing the urine become dark in color makes people who suffer from IgA disease susceptible to high levels of anxiety. IgA patients face loneliness, and young people who suffer from it become depressed.
- IgA is best confirmed after a biopsy.

- Life changes are necessary as patients begin to understand and accept that sometime in the future their kidneys might cease functioning. But the real killer is the suspense and the unpredictability of the disease.
- As the disease is a recent development, even nephrologists are unsure of its progress.

No major change was observed in Magda's health. She and her family went on vacations. She could attend her school, and her social life was not impaired. But her mind was held captive by her anxiety. Paolo would laugh it away. "*Que será, será*; whatever will be, will be! If it comes, we will manage it," he said, encouraging her.

Now, with thirty-one years living with IgA, Magda is able to accept her condition without any qualm. She faces some weakness, and her low hemoglobin has not yet been corrected by an EPO injection, which is used to treat anemia. Maybe in the future, being anemic could become a concern. Her creatinine fluctuates between 2.4 and 2.8; and her proteinuria fluctuates between 250 mg and 350 mg in twenty-four hours. Importantly, she has maintained the levels for the past ten years or more.

What did Magda do right? She was conscious of and strict with her diet, adopting a low-protein and low-salt vegetarian diet. She permitted herself an occasional treat with a small serving of meat. Though potassium was not a problem for her, her vegetables were partially leached. She had never consumed alcohol or smoked cigarettes, so taking narcotic drugs was something she didn't dream of. She had regular scheduled blood tests every three to six months and was diligent about taking medications for BP, cholesterol, and uric acid, including calcium, vitamins, and folic acid. Additionally, because fish oil was suggested as potentially good, Magda took a daily dose of it.

Early eating habits, inculcated by her mother, made Magda choose conservative diet plans. She avoided all packaged food with preservatives and sauces for fear of hidden salt. She included bread, cakes, and pasta in her diet, along with special renal foods that are low in sodium, potassium, phosphorus, and vegetable proteins. These incorporated rice, corn, and potatoes. She avoided desserts with eggs and cream.

None of these things were part of any renal diet recommended by her doctor.

Now Magda knows that at some point in her life, she will be brushed by the disease; it may even decide to live with her and be part of her life. Until then she will try to bring change to many lives.

Magda's Professional Growth and Knowledge Base
Magda's quest for information never ceases. Every opportunity to expand her portfolio, she grabs and takes it forward. In recent times, this has meant the formation of a children's group for IgA and HS purpura.

Following is a list of the Facebook groups for which Magda is administrator or coadministrator:

- Insufficienza renale cronica – IRC (CKD)
- Nefropatia IgA / Sindrome di Berger (Gromerulonefrite)
- Bambini & insufficienza renale

- IgA nephropathy
- Renal Patient Support Group
- Kidney Disease – Information updates
- Kids and Kidney Disease: Not Child's Play
- United Children Kidney Disease
- Mark's Private Kidney Group Page
- The Transplant Community Outreach
- Transplantados
- Nefropatia por IgA
- Children with IgA nephropathy & HS purpura

Three of these are Italian groups, one is based in Argentina, one is based in Spain or Latin America, one is based in the United Kingdom, and the others are based in the USA.

Magda is also editor of some renal magazines, for example, *Rein* écos and *Notizie dal mondo Associativo*. For more information, visit http://www.emodializzati.it/category/notizie-dal-mondo-associativo/.

Fresh news: On 22nd March Magada Bonacina received a kidney after becoming eligible for preventive kidney transplant.

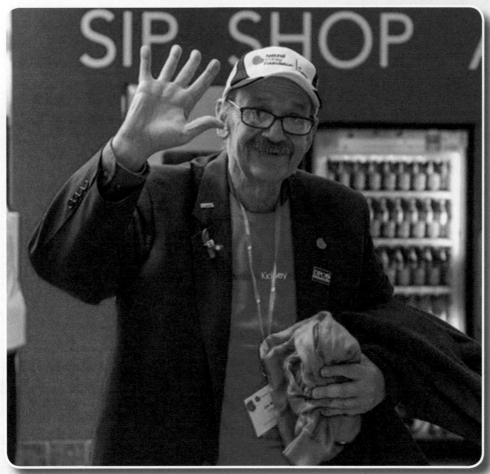

James Myers (Transplantee)

KIDNEY ADVOCACY RULES – JAMES MYERS

Young James grew up in a household with lots of mystery. There was always someone whispering down the long corridor. James would be puzzled. *Why are they talking so softly? They don't want me to hear?*

Then he would notice his uncle and his two aunts exchange strange looks that only they seemed to understand. His father would join them sometimes in such conversations. *So what are these secrets?*

As if they realized that James was puzzled, they would reach out to pat him briefly and then continue with their chats, looks, and nods, as if something big was being planned. Somehow he could sense there was some mystery. It was like a blanket of sorrow hanging so heavily that one could barely breathe fresh, clean air in their company.

But his mother was extremely sensitive to his needs. She treated him like a child who needed love. She would make extra efforts to cheer him up with her bright and cheerful chats.

As he grew up, he heard them talk about things like blood pressure. James could not make anything out of these discussions. But one day, the phrase *kidney disease* crept into the conversation, along with *BP, creatinine,* and *protein.* Now these became the new buzzwords. James began to follow the conversations with these words without understanding their significance.

When he questioned his mother, she explained to him that his father, uncles, and aunts were all suffering from a very serious kidney disease.

After some thought, he asked her, "So do I also have it, Mom?"

His mother hushed him, hugging him tightly, and asked him not to say such things. The way his mother had explained things made James appreciate his elders and be kind to them.

At times he would look around the house. *Everyone here is pretty sick!*

As he grew older, he began to feel it was normal for households to have such chats. Young James thought that because it had been so much a part of his life for so many years there was nothing abnormal about it. *But is it similar in other households?* James would wonder on his days off as he loitered in the corridor and then went off to study. At times he hated it all, and at other times he behaved as if he were above such chats and that none of them bothered him. One thing what struck him was that all his family members had an artificial smile painted on their sad faces. This was a façade, and they played it up, always hoping to make him feel better. Seeing them suffer, he would shrug his shoulders.

But the situation changed one day. When James Myers was twenty-five years old, polycystic kidney disease (PKD) became part of his life. It struck him like a thunderbolt. He became aware that he had jumped on the bandwagon of kidney patients in the family.

And then the scene changed in the family.

James's twenty-two-year-old cousin Rich died of kidney disease. That Rich was as young as James made the latter feel insecure. And he was very disturbed. One by one the other diseased elders, except his father, departed. So the house became shrouded in sorrow and pain.

No more were there whispers in the corridors, no more mystery in the air. Now the disease was very much around the house, in every nook and corner.

In 1983 his father began dialysis. Dialysis did not seem to go well for James's father, who was very uncomfortable and was really troubled by his dialysis sessions. James saw him suffer, and this added to his deep hurt and sorrow. Finally his father succumbed to CKD.

James became unsure. He wondered, *How will I live through this nightmare of a disease?*

In a quieter moment, with all earnestness, James decided to take a control of his health. He made many lifestyle changes, which seemed to be big sacrifices. But by ignoring those pangs of temptation, James managed to remain well for thirty-four years.

But things changed slowly. He could sense that his control was slipping. Small signs showed up. These were confirmed by the doctor to be bad signs.

"Jim, I think it's time to start your real treatment," the physician said with a little nod, his lips pursed, his eyes showing regret.

Preparation work for the fistula began making James very unhappy with the situation he had landed himself in. But he realized how important dialysis was for his health. So he settled down into his dialysis schedule. He also made time to get registered on three transplant lists. He needed a transplant. He constantly wondered, *When will I ever eat a slice of chocolate cake with no guilt attached? How I long for a hassle-free future without worrying about my kidney disease, simply enjoying life as it flows, and eating a complete meal without any restriction.*

Rolling his eyes, smacking his lips, he laughed at the mere thought of that joyous moment.

One day at the dialysis center, a friend was curious about how James had managed to remain away from dialysis for so long.

"Ah!" James said thoughtfully. "I just followed all the rules of the game. My physician told me to reduce a portion of my protein intake, add less salt to my food, and eat healthy meals with salad and fruits. So that was my diet." Mulling over how he'd lived the past few years, James continued. "I made regular visits to Indiana University Kidney Clinic to make sure my blood pressure was under control. I never missed medications. So my BP meds and diet were things I never lost sight of. I've been very strict with these two buddies all my years."

The friend rolled his eyes and said, "If only I knew dialysis could be postponed. I feel ashamed for being irregular with tests and medicines."

Another friend who had joined into the conversation asked James, "Jim, were you also working during this period?"

"Indeed, I was working as a trial lawyer, but eventually I couldn't be active, so I stopped working. But I was very lucky on two counts. I could work as a college professor and delay dialysis for a long time."

One day it occurred to him that this genetic condition could also affect the future generations. He spoke to his son. "Son, I need you to go through some tests, as polycystic kidney disease has already been with us for two generations. Let's see if you've inherited it as well."

It was the happiest day for James when his son's PKD tests were negative.

"Thank God we beat it!" he said, most thankfully.

James spent a few years on dialysis. Every day he posted on the Facebook, seeking a live kidney donor.

By April 2016, all his pretransplantation tests were completed. Finally James got "the call."

A lady spoke. "Hi, may I speak with James Myers?"

"Yes, this is James speaking."

That voice grew excited and said those magical words: "We have a kidney for you!"

James got his kidney, which he christened "Woody Woodrow."

All his life he'd been made intensely aware of kidney disease, and had fought it himself for many years. James got worked up when he realized that while the incidence of kidney disease was rising, there was not much awareness about the disease. Many people could have been saved with early detection if they had managed their blood pressure and diabetes. Polycystic kidney disease is an unavoidable genetic disease, but its progression can be slowed, which is also true for diabetes and hypertension.

James joined Facebook and opened several groups. There, along with many others, he would share important information. Slowly his advocacy work began. But he had a much larger contribution coming his way.

James shared with us how deeply he was aggrieved:

> When I was on dialysis, a law to cut funding to all dialysis centers was being proposed. It made me very angry. I looked around the room. All my clinic mates were too sick to fight back. I was the only one who had the energy in me, along with a strong sense of righteousness, to stop this law that could terminate many lives. So I acted.
>
> I joined several national organizations, including the National Kidney Foundation. I wrote several petitions and opinion editorials against the proposed law. I visited members of Congress in Washington, DC. I started to be more active online. Eventually, the law was defeated. I have been a kidney advocate ever since.

In 2015, James was honored with the National Social Media and Advocacy Award from the American Association of Kidney Patients. As part of the National Kidney Foundation, he is now the statewide advocate for the state of Indiana. James is a member of an elite group of advocates, the Kidney Advocacy Committee. He is a regional leader for Region #5 in the USA, consisting of the states of Michigan, Ohio, Indiana, Kentucky, and Tennessee. He meets advocates from those states to give advice and support.

James Myers is now waiting to go back to teaching. It is all about connecting with people with a story to tell.

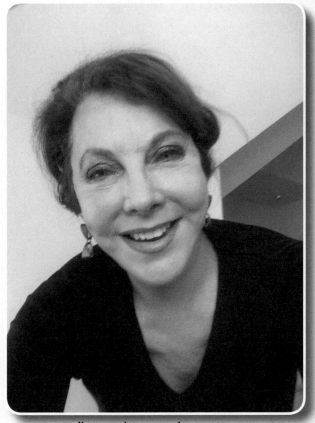

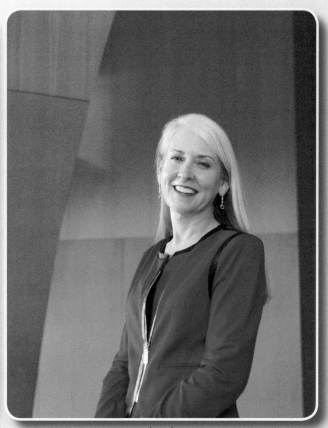

Sally Satel (Transplantee)

Virginia Postrel (Altruistic Donor)

ISN'T IT HIGH TIME TO REVIEW? – SALLY SATEL AND VIRGINIA POSTREL

I always felt that asking for a kidney was most difficult. But as I looked around, I found that altruistic kidney donors were gaining in popularity in the United States—something that should also happen in other countries!

One case that really inspired me was Sally Satel's story. The donor was Virginia Postrel, a renowned author and activist.

In November 2005 Virginia responded to Sally. "Serious offer" was the subject of the mail. The body read, "If I'm compatible, I'll be a donor. Best, Virginia."

She followed it two weeks later with, "By the way, I absolutely promise you that I will not back out."

On March 7, 2006, Virginia returned from the hospital feeling satisfied after the kidney was surgically transplanted. Read on for one of the most remarkable stories of organ donation.

Forty-nine-year-old Sally Satel, a psychiatrist and lecturer at the Yale University School of Medicine, resident scholar at the American Enterprise Institute, was diagnosed with failing kidneys in August

2004. Possibly it meant she could start dialysis six months down the line. No lifestyle condition like blood pressure or diabetes was evidenced at the onset of the disease. Nephrologists believed her condition could be the result of some medication she had taken nearly thirty years ago. It was an idiopathic kidney failure, a kind of glomerular disease.

Sally got herself listed on the national organ transplant list. She was sixty-one thousandth on the list at that time.

She did some investigating, studying data, and realized that it could be well over five years before she would be allotted a kidney for the transplant. She was not too comfortable with the thought of dialysis, which would alienate her from friends, not to mention the debilitating effects of the treatment. She had known of patients on dialysis experiencing cramps and vomiting spells and being confined to home.

Talking to friends and networking on the Web for a donor brought some positive results. Two friends almost handed over a kidney; some others tested and were not a good match. Seeking other avenues also meant registering with MatchingDonors.com. A result emerged when a sixty-two-year-old retired Canadian man responded to her request.

Sally was tentative at times, making him comfortable with his offer. They developed a rapport. His earnestness to be the donor became evident when he went to great lengths discussing logistics, including his insurance coverage and where and how to transplant the organ. All throughout that autumn she was engaged in active conversation, with a man promising an organ.

Through a mutual friend, Virginia had heard that Sally Satel was looking for a kidney donor. A few years ago the two women had interacted in a professional capacity on a project. So Virginia sent an offer in the mail. The Canadian's offer being still hot meant that another option for a donor was being pursued.

Sally had seen two friends move away on some pretext, but when the shutters were closed on the Canadian's offer, she was disheartened. Fortunately, Virginia's letter was comforting and gave her hope for relief. Virginia's letters expressed her intention to behave as a responsible donor, with a firm purpose to deliver.

Virginia went through the donor evaluation process and took the tests.

She was approved as a donor and the surgery took place.

Reflections
Why was Virginia Postrel so willing to part with an organ?

[Virginia, being "brazenly pragmatic," shared her take on donating a kidney: "I have a very instrumental view of my body, so when [Sally] needed a part, I was happy to give it."]

Virginia felt empathy and realized that since Sally had no family—her parents were dead and she had no sibling—she should help her constructively. It is this sentiment aroused in a person momentously that shows us how high some people's generosity can peak. Some hearts are simply made to be more caring.

To the world this story is unique.

There is no reason for Virginia's heartwarming gesture, but in Hindu philosophy it comes under the umbrella of what is popularly called "karma."

But the post-transplant scene opened a new way of thinking.

Surprisingly on this topic both Sally and Virginia exhibited the same line of thinking. For a kidney donor, the aura of heroism wanes as soon as the economics of the episode surface: the bills for travel and accommodations, and the loss of pay, puncture the sheer joy of giving when the financial reality surfaces. Kidney donors are not recognized for the sacrifices they make, nor does their heroic act give other people any great impetus to donate an organ.

Sally Satel has been fortunate to have had two friends each donate a kidney, one in 2006 and the second in 2016. The first transplant "galvanized me about the issue, not the surgery, but the process of finding a donor," she said on one occasion. This deep-seated anguish for humanity, at a vastly different level than commonly viewed, made her vocal about kidney transplants, with a new approach.

She analyzed the situation in the United States, as follows:

- Out of 120,000 people in need of an organ, 98,000 are waiting for a kidney transplant. The majority of them will have to wait for a deceased donor.
- "Twelve people will die tomorrow, by this time," she said, because they can't survive the wait. Every day twelve people on the list will die. It is indeterminate who will die first, as people's ends are determined by individual health condition, mental acceptance, and tolerance of the dialysis regimen.
- In 1984 the National Organ Transplant Act (NOTA) named altruism as the sole motivation for giving a kidney. If anyone were to accept valuable consideration, they could actually be prosecuted for a felony, facing a fine of $50,000 and/or five years' imprisonment.
- Many ways were consciously explored to increase the donor pool, including education about signing up for organ donation and special arrangements for emergency rooms to counsel families to release the organs of their beloved, among other things.
- Swap transplants were meant to be a great game-changer. It was indeed an excellent concept. But sadly the swap provided only five hundred new organs—compared to a requirement of ninety-eight thousand individuals!

Figure 2. Waiting time for a kidney

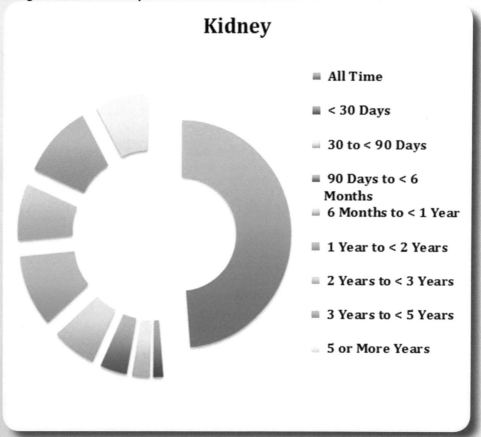

Kidney

- All Time
- < 30 Days
- 30 to < 90 Days
- 90 Days to < 6 Months
- 6 Months to < 1 Year
- 1 Year to < 2 Years
- 2 Years to < 3 Years
- 3 Years to < 5 Years
- 5 or More Years

Table developed by Vasundhara Raghavan.

In Sally's view, the ban on financial compensation is an obstacle to organ donation. While she categorically states she doesn't advocate for the "classic free market," she urges lawmakers to think of ways to incentivize potential donors. She suggests the following as a general outline of a model to reward people who help a stranger in this way:

- Tax forgiveness for expenses incurred for organ donation.
- Tax credits.
- Contribution to retirement account.
- Children's education voucher.
- Loan forgiveness.
- Donation to a charity of the person's choice.
- Consideration valued at about $50,000 that could come out of dialysis savings.
- On account of safeguarding dignity issues, there won't be any question of exploiting people from a low-income group.
- It can follow the first come, first served principle and take the usual time as with other transplants, which is about three months—enough time for a donor to come to understand the surgery and its implications and for the authorities to check if the person has been coerced.

Elaborating on her case for reviewing the existing system, she made some great observations, as follows:

"Our current transplant regime is a qualified failure. Transplant operations have been basically flat for the last eight years. In 2013, over forty-three hundred people died while waiting, and about three thousand were permanently removed from the queue because they developed a medical condition that precluded transplant. Twenty-seven years ago, the average wait for a deceased-donor kidney in the United States was about one year; now, the average wait is approaching five years. In many parts of the country it has reached a ten-year wait from listing to transplant—if one can survive that long."

Furthermore, Sally brings to memory strong words in support of compensation. But will this proposition find favor among people with a different outlook? A lesson in humanity and understanding the deep-rooted pain associated with chronic kidney disease is required.

"And, at one of the early NOTA hearings in the House, Al Gore, then the Tennessee congressman spearheading the legislation, spoke approvingly of 'the provision of incentives, such as a [presumably third party] voucher system or a tax credit to a donor's estate' if 'efforts to improve voluntary donation are unsuccessful.'"

But in the interests of the people who are struggling every other day to prepare mentally and physically for a session of dialysis, some drastic steps are much needed. Failure to react will wipe out communities of people with kidney disease as each year more people get recruited.

References:
See Restatement (Second) of Contracts § 71(1) (1979)
Copyright © 2014 by Sally Satel, Joshua C. Morrison, and Rick K. Jones, "State Organ-Donation Incentives Under the National Organ Transplant Act." This article is available at http://lcp.law.duke.edu/cgi/viewcontent.cgi?article=4699&context=lcp.

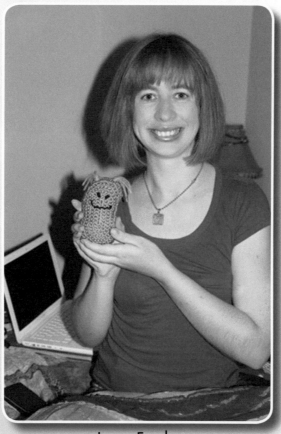

Jenna Franks

KIDNEYS FIND THEIR OWN
DESTINATION – JENNA FRANKS

Karol was reminiscing over her morning coffee about the long journey of finding kidneys for Jenna.

It was about small incidents that connected magically to help Jenna on two different occasions. The first incident, in 2006, was still quite fresh with regard to sensitivity. She was at her desk when she picked up the phone. The caller began, "Hi. I'm seeking some urgent information on crossmatch and antibodies …"

Karol was quick to pick up the cause for the caller's tension and explained how important it is to have lower level of antibodies so there's no risk to the transplanted kidney. During the conversation, she had suggested to the caller, Patrice Smith, that she check other prospects on the Living Donors waiting list.

Patrice gained her composure and went ahead to check the donor website.

What happened thereafter was a matter of pure coincidence. Patrice actually chose Jenna, Karol's twenty-one-year-old daughter, who was also looking for a kidney donor. The transplant happened much to the joy of the family.

But the life of that kidney was limited to seven years.

The second trip down the "organ search" lane had begun. Today, Karol can sigh, as this chapter has come to a close, but the days, months, and years leading up to it were filled with had many indelible moments.

At one point an email from Jenna's godmother had been very comforting.

That day it had played on Karol's mind as she carried through her work. At the dinner table, she had mentioned it. "Oh, by the way, today I had this amazing news from Rhonda. A few days ago, she had posted Jenna's story on her Facebook timeline, and her friend Gary Frey, a Marine veteran from Tucson, agreed to get tested for Jenna. He's offering her his kidney!"

"That's good news!" her husband Ed said eagerly.

Though the news created some buzz around the table, with Jenna, James, Becca, and Johnny talking excitedly, Karol added tentatively, "But we need to do the tests before jumping to any conclusions."

Though the topic was put to rest, there was some renewed hope for Jenna. For a second transplant she needed a good live donor match. Her body's rejection of the previous transplant had left Jenna with a very high level of antibodies, making it very difficult to find a match. Statistically, out of ten thousand, only three people could be her perfect match. So what was the probability that Gary Frey was one of these three?

A string of emails from Rhonda and Gary kept the topic hot enough for Jenna's family to pursue the matter and get the tests done. To have a dialogue with a willing donor was really a blessing, as many people on Facebook were looking for a donor.

In a few weeks, however, it was confirmed. Gary was a good candidate, but he was not a match for Jenna.

Over the years, many friends, family members, and strangers tested, with no success.

But Jenna was not one to keep quiet. Together, she and Gary joined a kidney-pairing donation program called the National Kidney Registry, a transplant option for prospective recipients who had a willing but incompatible donor. The only way for Gary to donate to a recipient was for there to be a suitable match for Jenna, but no match had been found since she'd registered for the program.

Surprisingly Gary stayed committed for five years.

Finally the big day arrived. Gary's kidney was transplanted on July 18, 2017.

With Gary giving away his kidney, the transplant team at UCLA began working on Jenna's antibodies with treatments of Rituximab, plasmapheresis, thymoglobulin, and intravenous immunoglobulin (IVIg). Then the wait-and-watch game for the right match began.

This period was spiked with worry and planning, with high-riding faith that good luck would knock at Jenna's door soon. There was a huge amount of suspense built around the timing of when the donor would show up. Things were still not completely under Jenna's control. She went through each day with great expectations. Hopefully an organ would be found.

And then … hurray. The moment had arrived. In Karol's words, "Call it coincidence or fate, or thanks to Gary's good karma, Jenna got a call from the UCLA transplant team, saying that the National Kidney Registry had found a compatible match for Jenna!"

Being that the person was a swap donor, the family was not given many details. But the joy of its being Jenna's first call in five years was heartwarming.

Jenna started desensitization treatments. These showed a considerable decrease in her very high antibodies.

On July 26, 2017, a kidney from an anonymous donor was flown from the northeast United States to Los Angeles, and Jenna had her transplant surgery. Throughout the surgery, messages were posted to social media. There were updates and lots of kind inquiries to be responded to. Lots of wishes and prayers came pouring in, so the family was truly overwhelmed.

Karol recalled the few quiet moments in the hospital.

She had looked at her thirty-one-year-old daughter Jenna as she was recovering. What a tough time it had been for Jenna since her high school days. The initial shock that she and her family felt when she was diagnosed with a rare urological defect that was silently destroying her kidneys was huge. Karol thought of how inconvenient it was, when there were young girls and boys having a great time. Even while in high school, Jenna had been on dialysis. For three years she had continued with this treatment.

Then phenomenal things had happened.

Karol felt her heart fill with gratitude for the fact that in 2012, Rhonda had posted about Jenna needing a donor and Gary decided to commit to donate.

Karol wondered what had allowed him to wait so long, never considering going back on his promise. It spoke volumes of his humanity and his singular purpose to do an altruistic act. In her heart, the love and respect for Gary rose to a peak. Gary had entered their lives and left a huge treasure, one that was priceless.

Jenna's treatments—plasmapheresis, IVIg, and antithymocyte globulin—will be ongoing, to reduce antibodies to protect her from rejecting the organ. She will be on immunosuppressive medications for the life of the transplanted kidney.

***

The aspect of uncovered expenses for the donor has always been a problem in live donor transplants. A donor's medical expenses are basically covered by insurance, but the donor needs to meet expenses for travel and lodging, and make up for lost wages for time taken off for testing, surgery, and recovery. Federal law prohibits the sale of an organ, but an exception is allowed for "reasonable payments" for those expenses incurred by a living kidney donor. A GoFundMe campaign was started in this case.

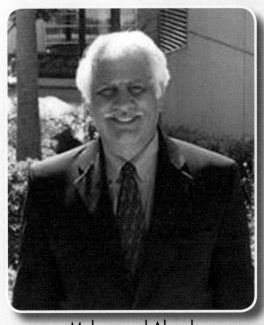

Mohammad Akmal

SELF-DIAGNOSING MY KIDNEY CANCER – MOHAMMAD AKMAL

It is very normal for me to wake up sometime in between sleep to visit the toilet. But two years ago I had a shocking experience. At 2am even though my eyes were heavy with sleep I noticed flank blood in my urine. The nephrologist in me was fully awake and raised questions, "No pain in the kidney, so is it what I suspect?" I went back to bed and shared my new worry with my wife, "I think I may have a kidney cancer!"

She stirred in bed and responded in a sleepy voice, " What makes you make this comment at this unearthly hour?"

"I just passed blood in the urine and I have no pain. Painless hematuria suggests that it could be kidney cancer!"

I visited my physician next morning requesting for an ultra sound of the kidneys. It showed some swelling of the ureter (left hydroureter). I made a quick mental note, "I must get to the bottom of this!" but with a medical conference in New York I was busy the whole week.

Another episode of bloody urine while returning to California became a cause for worry and eventually I decided to focus on my health. Visiting a local hospital in the Bay Area I managed to get an abdomen CT scan done. It revealed a left hydroureter with a tumor that was more than 3 cms in size. Years' of experience helped me conclude that it was transitional cell carcinoma. But I knew it had to be backed with a biopsy.

I headed to an urologist for a biopsy unfortunately he couldn't accomplish the task, as it was difficult to pass the stent to reach the tumor. So the biopsy was halted.

When finally the biopsy of the tumor was managed, the diagnosis was confirmed as transitional cell carcinoma. A team of urologists recommended removal of the left kidney, left ureter and evaluate the pelvis area of the urinary bladder.

Before my surgery I underwent another round of tests including a CT scan, MRI and PET scan and the relevant blood tests. These tests showed that the disease was limited to the ureter though some insignificant activity was seen in the pelvis.

A robotic surgery that lasted 14 hours was performed to remove the affected kidney and left ureter. It was longer than usual because of adhesions from previous surgery. After a successful surgery I was discharged after about 5 days stay at the hospital. My postoperative course was excellent.

A few months later, my first surveillance was uneventful. My surgeon congratulated me saying, "It is one of the rare occasions that I can tell the patient *you are cured from this cancer.*"

I can sadly say, cancer is like a chameleon and it can fool us at any time. It resurfaced a few months later putting me on a tough road of recovery.

My second diagnostic imaging showed a new lesion in the previously located kidney area. I approached a general surgeon requesting him to remove the lesion by an open abdominal surgery.

In a pre surgery evaluation, some glands were detected in my left neck. Suspecting it to be a second cancer an ultrasound of my neck was done followed by a biopsy of the glands. The tests confirmed it was cancer and so the line of treatment changed.

I was subjected to powerful chemotherapy that I didn't tolerate well.

I felt these 6 months of life was my most miserable period in life, as I needed to handle so many complications. Such as the frequent nausea and vomiting episodes, irritation caused by lack of appetite, generalized skin rash, peripheral neuropathy (dead feeling and numbness), weakness of muscles, fatigue, frequent falls and most annoying aspect was my disturbed sleep.

But suddenly some good fortune came my way. During this period immunotherapy was approved in the USA for treatment and many people benefited from it. Doctors were kind enough to offer me immunotherapy, which was intravenously administered once in every 3 weeks. As soon as immunotherapy was initiated, my life miraculously changed. My cancer gradually seemed to be under control. I feel so grateful to God that I was given a second chance to live.

Today I'm able to laugh it away, but there are times when I sit and reflect on what had transpired. It is ironic how a nephrologist who treated so many patients, faced some kind of kidney disease. I also think of how each of my patients' would have faced their life challenging experiences. Now I feel I am in a better position to treat patients by fully appreciating their feelings as I am on their side of the fence.

(Mohammad Akmal is author, nephrologist and kidney-cancer survivor)

PART II: MEDICAL FACTS AND EMOTIONAL SUPPORT

Our purpose for adding some pertinent information on the medical aspects of kidney disease is to offer guidance and information. Some information about the disease appears in the foregoing narratives, but more detailed information provided by an experienced nephrologist is found in this section. For more in-depth information, you might like to read nephrology journals and medical books.

This section includes the following chapters:

- Many Conditions That Could Lead to Kidney Failure, by Dr. Mohammad Akmal
- CKD Management, Issues, and Treatments, by Dr. Mohammad Akmal
- Safe Pregnancy for the Patient and the Unborn, by Dr. Mohammad Akmal
- Patient-Centric Aspects: Trauma and the Need for Support, by Vasundhara Raghavan
- The Ride beyond Rejection, by Vasundhara Raghavan
- Facing Kidney Failure, by Vasundhara Raghavan

MANY CONDITIONS THAT COULD
LEAD TO KIDNEY FAILURE

Dr. Mohammad Akmal

Diabetes and hypertension are recognized as two of the most common secondary reasons for kidney failure. Kidney failure is related to such preexisting conditions.

Taking Guard
It is established and recognized worldwide that since both diabetes and hypertension could end in a kidney failure, early preventive action is extremely advisable to prevent either one, or both, from leading to a kidney failure. Periodic blood tests and blood pressure checks, coupled with controlling diet and getting regular exercise, will change the way the future will pan out for patients with diabetes and blood pressure.

Diabetes as Related to Kidney Failure
In my association with patients, I have met many who have courageously met the new challenge of having kidney disease. These people need special mention. But it would be useful first to briefly discuss diabetes-related kidney disease.

Diabetes is a condition in which the patient has an elevated blood sugar level either because the body does not produce sufficient insulin or the body cells do not respond to the insulin produced. Insulin, the hormone produced by the pancreas, enables the body cells to absorb glucose to turn it into energy. The definition of diabetes mellitus was recently modified by the American Diabetes Association to include several independent criteria to establish the diagnosis, such as a 75 g oral glucose tolerance test with a 2-h value of 200 mg/dL, or more, a random plasma glucose of 200 mg/dL, or more with typical symptoms of diabetes and a fasting glucose of 126 mg/dL or greater on more than one occasion. Fasting glucose values are preferred for their convenience and reproducibility. There are many types of diabetes, the most common of which are as follows:

- Type 1 – Failure of the body to produce insulin.
- Type 2 – Cells fail to use insulin properly, sometimes combined with an insulin deficiency.
- Gestational – When a pregnant woman who never had diabetes before develops high blood glucose levels during pregnancy. It may eventually result in type 2 diabetes.

As of 2000, at least 171 million people worldwide suffer from diabetes, 2.8% of the population. Its incidence is increasing rapidly, and the number is expected to double by 2030. (Recent information provided by the International Diabetes Federation, Brussels, Belgium, gives an estimate of 250 million as of November 2008. Unless deliberate measures are taken by 2030, the incidence will be much higher.)

In 2008 the number of diabetics in the USA was 24 million; of those, 5.7 million remain undiagnosed. Another 57 million individuals are estimated to be prediabetic, and an additional 30 million to 40 million people are believed to have impaired glucose tolerance, resulting in health care costs exceeding

$100 billion annually. Of the two types, type 2 affects 90%–95%, and 5%–10% of the US diabetic population suffers from type 1.

The prevalence of diabetes increases with age. This is supported by real estimates that show 18.3% (8.6 million) of Americans above sixty years old are diabetic. Approximately 20%–30% of diabetics will develop kidney disease, and about half of the patients who started dialysis are diabetics (a greater percentage with type 2, which has a higher base).

Type 2 diabetes is more common in Native Americans, Hispanics, African Americans, Asians, and Pacific Islanders, as compared to Caucasians. The increased incidence in developing countries is partly the result of increased urbanization and adopting a Western lifestyle, particularly when it comes to diet. Another emerging group is young people facing obesity, who are hence more prone to developing the disease. Besides being potential diabetics, other contributory factors such as high blood pressure, poor control of diabetes, focal segmental glomerulonephritis, lipid abnormalities, and smoking put this age group at higher risk of developing chronic kidney disease (CKD).

Diabetics with CKD carry poor prognosis, as those on dialysis or those who are recipients of a kidney transplant are faced with increased morbidity and mortality due to coexistent diabetic complications. Poor vision, heart disease, circulatory insufficiency, nerve damage, and amputations are additional problems contributing to the misery of these patients. Reports show that more than half of the patients die within two years of initiating dialysis.

How Does a Person Know That He or She Is Diabetic?

A person with diabetes experiences one or more of the telltale symptoms. Once any of these symptoms are noticed, the person can seek doctor's help, and necessary medications can be taken to control diabetes. The symptoms are as follows:

- blurred vision
- frequent urination
- increased thirst
- weight loss
- slow-healing sores
- feelings of hunger and tiredness

Diabetes is a long-term disease that has no cure, but with careful control of blood sugar, complications of the disease can be delayed or prevented. It is important to note, however, that many people have no signs or symptoms before they are diagnosed with diabetes.

Hypertension
Hypertension, a common chronic medical condition, follows diabetes as the second common cause of CKD. In the sixth century BC, the writings of Sushruta Samhita (a Sanskrit interpretation of Ayurvedic concepts) first mentioned symptoms like those of hypertension. The modern understanding of hypertension began with the work of physician William Harvey (1578–1657), and a century later

Richard Bright recognized hypertension as a disease entity. Frederick Mahomed (1849–1884) was the first to report high blood pressure in a patient without kidney disease.

Locating the Reason for High Blood Pressure

As part of its function, the heart pumps blood into the arteries, which carry blood to all parts of the body. Blood pressure (BP) is the measured force of the blood as it hits the walls of the arteries. Normal blood pressure is 120 (systolic reading) when the heart pumps and 80 (diastolic reading) when the heart rests.

According to the National Heart, Lung, and Blood Institute (NHLBI), high blood pressure (HBP) is a reading of blood pressure of 140/90 mm Hg or higher. Both the numbers forming the range are important for assessment of blood pressure. Once a person develops HBP, it generally lasts a lifetime.

Hypertension is classified either as essential (no known medical cause) or secondary (the result of another cause, such as kidney disease, renal artery stenosis, adrenal tumor, or pheochromocytoma).

A recent classification brings clarity to the condition:

Classification	Systolic blood pressure (in mm Hg)	Diastolic blood pressure (in mm Hg)
Normal	90–119	60–79
Prehypertension	120–139	80–89
Stage 1 hypertension	140–159	90–99
Stage 2 hypertension	> 160	> 100
Isolated systolic hypertension	> 140	< 90

An adult is known to be hypertensive if his or her BP is high on two or more BP readings, obtained more than one minute apart at two or more office visits. (Note that BP after smoking, eating, and/or consuming caffeinated beverages will be elevated, so the BP must be measured after an hour of such activity, particularly after eating salty foods.)

Physicians specializing in hypertension conduct twenty-four-hour ambulatory BP monitoring before establishing the case as hypertension. Under this monitoring, multiple BP readings over a prolonged period of time are obtained. Complete understanding of the condition is possible if the collected information is assessed by the following parameters:

- mean twenty-four-hour BP
- mean daytime BP
- mean nighttime BP
- average difference between waking and sleeping BP
- evaluation of nocturnal dipping (a decrease in mean arterial BP of more than 10% during sleep)
- above other variations in BP

As in adults, blood pressure in children is variable between individuals, within individuals, by day, and at different times of the day. Studies show the distribution of patients with hypertension as follows:

- Preadolescents – 60%–70% is of secondary type and renal parenchymal disease.
- Adolescents – 80%–90% is largely the essential type.
- Adults – 90%–95% is the essential type. Among people with secondary hypertension it is known that primary hyperaldosteronism is the most frequent endocrine form. Hypertension is frequently part of metabolic X syndrome, which also includes diabetes, dyslipidemia, and central obesity.

Blood pressure is usually measured with a *sphygmomanometer* during a visit to the doctor, though sometimes it may be done at home by patients. The device derives its name from the Greek word *sphygmós*, which means "pulse," combined with a scientific term for "pressure meter," *manometer.*

Knowing the Condition
More than 90% of BP patients have essential hypertension, while the other 10% of cases have secondary hypertension. This is how the patients are evaluated in the primary care setting.

Essential hypertension is a heterogeneous and polygenic condition resulting from dysregulation of hormones, proteins, and neurogenic factors involved in BP regulation. Dietary factors and inactivity largely contribute to an increase in incidence. Impaired loss of salt by the kidneys plays a pivotal role in the pathogenesis of hypertension. Although 30% to 60% of BP variability is inherited, the common gene that significantly affects BP is yet to be identified.

Polymorphism in alleles at many different loci interacts with behavioral and environmental factors, resulting in the final disease trait. Rare monogenic forms of hypertension have also been identified. Nearly all genes identified playing a role in the pathogenesis of hypertension cause changes in salt handling by the kidneys, thus providing credence to the importance of excretion of sodium by the kidneys in the development of hypertension.

Secondary hypertension is most commonly caused by kidney disease, primary hyperaldosteronism, renovascular disease, or pheochromocytoma.

Other causes include endocrine dysfunction or exogenous factors like oral contraceptives, nonsteroidal anti-inflammatory drugs (NSAIDs), erythropoietin (used to correct anemia in patients with renal failure and cancer), calcineurin inhibitors (e.g., cyclosporine and Prograf) used for organ transplantation, and sympathomimetic agents (catecholamines, epinephrine, norepinephrine, and dopamine).

Patients who have atypical clinical features and are resistant* to therapy for BP control may be considered to have secondary hypertension. This should be the guiding factor for adopting the line of treatment.

Narrowing Hypertension Type to Determine Treatment
Apart from essential and secondary, further types of hypertension should be identified and determined. Understanding and eliminating these types will bring clarity when treating the condition.

Resistant hypertension is characterized by failure to achieve a target BP control with optimal dosages of three different class of BP medications, including a diuretic. With this type, it is difficult to determine if a person is resistant. If a person is noncompliant with medications, leading to poor BP control, it would be wrong to conclude that the person is resistant to therapy when the therapy has been inadequate.

The predisposing factors associated with resistant hypertension include the following:

- older age
- black ethnicity
- obesity (BMI > 30)
- diabetes underlying hypertension
- drugs that may increase BP (cocaine, NSAIDs, cyclosporine, and erythropoietin, e.g.), excessive alcohol consumption, and increased intake of sodium

Before concluding that the person is resistant, factors like obesity, sleep apnea, and secondary types of hypertension (primary aldosteronism and renovascular hypertension) should be considered and ruled out.

About 50%–60% of patients with sleep apnea are affected by hypertension, and conversely about 50% of patients with hypertension have sleep apnea. A strong association is particularly found in patients with resistant hypertension and usually results from excessive salt intake, nocturnal hypoxemia-mediated sustained elevated sympathetic nervous system activity, excessive aldosteronism, and obesity associated with insulin resistance.

A smaller percentage of cases may be found to be white coat hypertension, masked hypertension, or exercise-induced hypertension.

People who are noticed to have high blood pressure in the doctor's office are said to have white coat hypertension. This kind of hypertension is defined by BP measurements above 140/90 mm Hg during at least during separate visits to the doctor's office and with at least two sets of measurements below 140/90 mm Hg in nonclinical settings, in the absence of target organ damage. Some people experience "lab coat syndrome," defined by skyrocketing BP when approached by a medical professional wearing a stethoscope.

The ambulatory BP measurement is considered to be the gold standard for detecting patients who have resistant hypertension and differentiating them from those with white coat hypertension. This involves checking BP regularly, and taking readings at home and/or at work to estimate the average BP measurements in day-to-day real-life situations.

Patients with white coat hypertension have a lower risk of cardiovascular disease as compared to those with sustained hypertension. Though these patients have a greater tendency to develop sustained hypertension, pharmacologic treatment of white coat hypertension has not been shown to decrease morbidity.

Masked hypertension is characterized by a normal office BP but a high ambulatory BP measurement.

This condition appears to affect about ten million people in the United States and definitely carries a higher risk for cardiovascular disease when compared to those with normal office and ambulatory BP measurements. Treatment may begin if ambulatory BP measurements are elevated but there are no clinical trials available for the treatment of masked hypertension.

Exercise-induced hypertension is characterized by the presence of systolic BP of at least 186 mm Hg in African American men, 182 mm Hg in white men, 174 mm Hg in African American women, and 162 mm Hg in white women. The upper normal systolic values during exercise reach levels between 200 and 230 mm Hg. The prevalence of left-ventricular hypertrophy in these patients is 33% compared to others. Among these patients, the prevalence of a low ankle-brachial index is about 40%, compared to 18% in others. People with exercise-induced hypertension may demonstrate a greater amount of carotid plaque and a larger left ventricular mass but do not show abnormalities in the exercise ECG or thallium scan. These people appear to have an increased risk of peripheral vascular disease, carotid disease, and left ventricular hypertrophy, and exercise-induced hypertension may be a precursor marker of significant vascular disease. Those with exercise-induced hypertension should be treated with aggressive cardiovascular risk-reduction therapy that should include measures to reduce lipids and blood pressure.

How to Manage and Treat Hypertension
Management of hypertension includes lifestyle modifications and drug treatment for all patients with stage 1 or greater hypertension. The goal should be to decrease BP below 140/90 mm Hg, a measurement that is universally applicable for all hypertension patients.

Lifestyle modifications include weight reduction, a DASH diet (rich in fruits, vegetables, and low-fat dairy products, with a reduced content of saturated and total fat), reduction of sodium intake below 2.4 g every twenty-four hours, aerobic physical activity for thirty to thirty-four minutes most days, and limited daily alcohol consumption to two drinks for men and one drink for women.

If single-agent antihypertensive therapy is not effective within one to three months of treatment, the consulting doctor should be informed. A change in medication or adding a drug with a complementary mechanism of action may be advised.

Resistant hypertension should be managed by making lifestyle modifications, stopping the medications that may increase BP, and correcting the secondary causes. Resistant hypertension is usually associated with volume expansion and requires diuretic therapy.

Patients with sleep apnea should receive appropriate treatment with continuous positive airway pressure (CPAP).

In all cases of secondary hypertension, the cause should be identified and treated aggressively.

Generally, it is hard to establish whether kidney failure is due to high BP or due to kidney disease. However, essential hypertension is responsible for more than 90% of cases, and a good history, nature of previous follow-ups, and appropriate diagnostic evaluation may help in establishing the correct diagnosis.

Finally, the cause of hypertension is predominantly unknown. It is prudent to rule out secondary causes, because treatment of some of these conditions may provide a permanent cure of hypertension. Unfortunately, inadequate measures in the diagnosis of hypertension and its poor control result in enormous human, economic, and medical costs to society.

Hypertension in Combination with Diabetes
In patients with diabetes, hypertension adds significantly to the risk of vascular disease and death. It is recommended that hypertension in these patients be aggressively controlled and that BP be kept below 130/90 mm Hg. In most patients with diabetes, it is found that two or more antihypertensive agents are required to achieve the target BP control.

Uncontrolled BP affects a person adversely.

A person with high BP must get it treated and controlled, as this disease could put the person at great health risk. The health problems that may surface are as follows:

- cardiovascular disease, such as angina, stroke, and heart attack
- kidney damage
- damaged eyesight

High blood pressure can damage the blood vessels in the kidney, which could mean that wastes and excess fluid do not get removed. The excess fluid will increase the blood pressure, and over time if a person does little to lower the blood pressure through diet and medication, this may lead to kidney failure.

This causes a condition called *nephrosclerosis*.

Other Causes of Kidney Failure
The primary reasons for kidney failure are inherent problems with the kidney that could at times be genetic. It may be noted that an individual has no control over the disease and its progress. Hence it is a natural consequence of the state of the organ. Some of the causes of kidney disease are as follows:

- glomerular nephritis
- IgA nephropathy
- polycystic kidney disease
- Alport syndrome
- reflux nephropathy
- kidney stones and infection
- chronic interstitial nephritis
- chronic renal failure
- vasculitis
- kidney cancer
- lupus

There are many other very rare diseases, like atypical hemolytic uremic syndrome (aHUS), neurogenic bladder, spina bifida, primary hyperoxaluria, and hypophosphatemic rickets, and new conditions are emerging each day.

Glomerular Nephritis
This is one of the most common causes of kidney disease. Diseases may affect kidney function when they attack the *glomeruli* (tiny units in the kidney that clean blood). Glomerular diseases could be caused by genetics or environmental factors, but they largely fall in to the following two categories:

- glomerulonephritis – inflammation of the membrane tissue that acts as a filter, separating the waste and extra fluid from the blood
- glomerulosclerosis – when tiny blood vessels in the kidney are scarred or become hardened

Both these conditions lead to kidney failure. The majority of cases are the result of the formation of antibodies to *glomeruli* or the filtering of antigen-antibody complexes by glomeruli.

The diseases damage the glomeruli, and in the process some protein and red blood cells leak into the urine. The kidneys normally clear these waste products. Sometimes this filtration may be affected so that waste is left in the blood. The loss of blood protein such as albumin indicates a drop in the level of albumin in the blood. Albumin plays a vital role in absorbing extra fluid from the body into the bloodstream, until the kidney finally removes the extra fluid. Due to the lower level of albumin, the capacity to absorb the excess fluid is reduced. Excess fluid is retained, which could lead to swelling in the face, hands, feet, or ankles.

Common Signs of Glomerular Disease

Before being checked up by a doctor, you can detect glomerular disease by noting the following:

- The urine is frothy, indicating high levels of protein in the urine.
- The urine is pinkish in color, which could be blood in the urine.
- There is swelling in parts of the body, which is called *edema*.

Blood tests could reveal the following:

- low blood protein, in medical terms, *hypoproteinemia*
- high levels of creatinine, urea, and nitrogen in the blood, indicating that the kidneys' capacity to filter waste is affected, which is known as *reduced glomerular filtration*

Urine analysis could show the following:

- high levels of protein – *proteinuria*
- blood in the urine – *hematuria*

If both the blood and urine tests show some signs of the above problems, a *renal imaging* ultrasound or x-ray may be recommended. Other than this, a kidney biopsy may help in confirming glomerular disease and identifying the exact reason for the disease.

Known Causes of Glomerular Disease

There are a number of different diseases that could result in swelling or scarring of the nephron or glomerulus, leading to glomerular disease. These causes include infection, a drug that harms kidneys, or a disease like *diabetes* or *lupus* that affects the entire body. Sometimes glomerular disease can occur without reason or without being associated with any disease.

IgA Nephropathy

Many names have been derived from the description of kidney changes observed by kidney biopsy over three decades, but IgA nephropathy is the name commonly used. Berger's disease was often used in the past to describe the currently known IgA nephropathy. Berger's disease was named after a French pathologist, Jean Berger, who first reported seminal observations in Paris in the late 1960s.

IgA neuropathy is the response of the immune system to viruses. This response affects the kidneys. When the body is attacked, it releases *immunoglobulin A (IgA)*, a protein that helps the body fight infections. Sometimes the IgA protein gets stuck in the kidneys, resulting in inflammation. With this inflammation comes blood (hematuria) and protein (proteinuria) in the urine. A biopsy is needed to confirm the disease.

IgA is most often a slowly progressive disease, so people can manage the disease for a long time, though in some people it grows aggressively, leading to kidney failure. Some instances have been found where the disease has affected a cluster of families. There could be genetic factors playing a role in spreading the disease.

Polycystic Kidney Disease

Polycystic kidney disease (PKD) is a genetic disorder. It is caused by cysts in the kidney that are water filled. PKD cysts enlarge the kidneys, thereby replacing much of the normal structure, resulting in reduced kidney function and leading to kidney failure.

After a few years in cases when PKD results in kidney failure, the person will require dialysis or kidney transplantation. With the most common type of PKD, about half the patients suffer kidney failure.

PKD can cause cysts in the liver and create problems for blood vessels in the brain and heart. To determine if this is a case of PKD or a simple cyst, information on the number of cysts and the complications they cause is sufficient.

Alport Syndrome

Alport syndrome, the second most common inherited cause of kidney failure, usually affects young men. It can affect older people and women, too.

In each kidney there are one million tiny filtering units (glomeruli), and blood is filtered across the glomerular basement membrane (GBM). In Alport syndrome, one of the proteins that make up the

GBM is absent or abnormal. The GBM looks normal in childhood, but it deteriorates over time because it lacks the special protein. This leads to kidney failure. This basement membrane is also found in the inner ears and in parts of the eyes, which means that Alport syndrome could lead to deafness and eye problems.

Alport syndrome is much more common in boys and men, as the gene that usually causes it (called COL4A5) is on the X chromosome. Men have only one X chromosome, whereas women have two X chromosomes (XX), so women usually have a normal copy as well as an abnormal copy of the gene.

Women who carry the disease may have minor kidney trouble, such as blood or protein in the urine, sometimes with high blood pressure, but occasionally they do develop a severe disease and kidney failure. The lifetime risk of severe kidney disease for women who carry Alport syndrome may be as high as one in five, but most never have severe trouble, and those who do are usually much older than men who are affected.

Chronic Interstitial Nephritis

When the spaces between the kidney tubules become swollen or inflamed, they can affect the kidney's ability to filter the waste products. This condition is called interstitial nephritis. If this is a short-term condition, it is acute. It may become worse and develop into a chronic condition.

Some of the causes for interstitial nephritis could be the following:

- drug allergies
- analgesic nephropathy caused by damage to the kidney due to prolonged use of pain relievers
- effects of certain antibiotics
- medications such as nonsteroidal anti-inflammatory drugs (NSAIDs), furosemide, and thiazide diuretics

When interstitial nephritis becomes severe, it is likely to be chronic and damage the kidneys, particularly in elderly patients.

Some symptoms that may be noticed are the following:

- blood in the urine
- change in volume of urine output
- change in mental condition, such as feeling drowsy or confused
- feeling of nausea
- rashes
- swelling
- weight gain due to fluid retention

Chronic Renal Failure

Chronic renal failure (CRF) occurs when some large blood vessels have abnormalities. If a renal artery is narrowed by stenosis, the large arteries are unable to supply adequate blood to the kidneys for their functioning. This leads to elevated blood pressure, resulting in hypertension. Insufficient blood supply could shrink the kidney and result ultimately in a CRF.

Vasculitis

This is an inflammation of the small blood vessels and covers many uncommon diseases involving the vascular system. In vasculitis, the inflammation damages the walls of various blood vessels. A certain pattern is involved in the distribution of blood vessels and how they reach particular organs. Through tests abnormalities are revealed. The organ that will be affected by the blood vessel is determined by which organ is reached by the blood vessel. As a group, these diseases are referred to as vasculitides.

Kidney Cancer

Renal cancer (kidney cancer) is caused by the kidneys' cells becoming cancerous and growing into a tumor. In most people, kidney cancer is seen in the linings of the kidneys' tiny tubes (tubules). Most kidney cancers are detected when they metastasize to distant organs. Early detection always makes it easier to treat kidney cancer successfully. However, these tumors could grow large before the cancer is discovered.

Renal cancer was first reported in 1826. Scientists have yet to discover its cause. Kidney cancer occurs most often after the age of forty; however, children as young as six months have been diagnosed. Kidney cancer affects almost twice as many men as women. It also tends to be somewhat more common in African American men than white men.

Overall, the lifetime risk for developing kidney cancer is about 1 in 63 (1.6%).

Lupus

Lupus as a disorder was noticed in three periods, classical, neoclassical, and modern. The disease was recognized in the Middle Ages (the classical period) as a classic malar rash and was referred to as lupus, a description given by the twelfth-century physician Rogerius. The neoclassical period of lupus began in 1872 with Móric Kaposi's revealing the systemic manifestations of the disease. Discovery of the LE (lupus erythematosus) cells in 1948 heralded the modern period. LE cells, however, are also found in other conditions. The disease is now characterized by advances in the knowledge of the pathophysiology, clinical and laboratory features, and treatment.

The Condition

Lupus nephropathy or systemic lupus erythematosus (SLE) is a rheumatic disease in which autoantibodies are directed against self-antigens, immune complex formation, and immune dysregulation. The disease's manifestations are adequately explained by the disease's name. *Systemic* describes the capability of the disease to affect many organs or systems in the body, involving both internal and external parts of the body. The rash that appears with the onset of the disease covers the cheeks and the bridge of the nose. This coverage reminds doctors of the wolf's white patch on its face. In Latin the word for "wolf" is *lupus*, which is how the disease got its name. Lastly, *erythematosus* means "red" in Latin, which is color of the skin rash brought about by lupus.

The illness is recognized as being unpredictable, with patients exhibiting symptoms of or being affected by the acute life-threatening disease. Because of its protean manifestations, lupus should be diagnosed by its differing conditions, such as fevers whose origin cannot be established, anemia, some types of nephritis, psychosis, arthralgia, and even fatigue. Patients being diagnosed early and receiving treatment for their symptoms has helped in the prognosis of this disease that was earlier considered to be fatal.

The disease affects the immune system, which has millions of white blood cells that protect the body from foreign invasions, such as by bugs or germs, thereby guarding against infections. The white blood cells are grouped according to specific tasks assigned in fighting invaders or foreign antigens. A population of cells called monocytes have the capability of recognizing foreign antigens and sending alerts to the T cells or T lymphocytes, which help in fighting the antigens. In turn the T cells send a message to the B lymphocytes, which produce the antibodies that overpower the antigens by attaching to them.

The cells eat up the antigen/antibody complexes, thereby cleaning up the mess. When sufficient antibodies are produced to counter the antigens, further production of antibodies is stopped by a signal sent to suppressor T cells, that is, another group of T cells. Finally the communication is received by B cells to stop the production activity. In the healthy immune system, things return to normal until the next time the person gets sick.

The Symptoms and the Causes

In a person with lupus, the immune system does not work properly for an unidentified reason. The antibodies produced by B cells attack the antigens, but the antigens in this case are not foreign invaders but parts of the person's body, either cells or tissues. So a person diseased by lupus makes autoantibodies that react with self-antigens, and these two combine to make immune complexes.

Cells assigned with the cleaning task clean up the immune complexes circulated by the blood. But over time, cleaning immune complexes becomes a huge challenge and the cells tire from the activity. The immune complexes travel with the blood vessels, and on the way they are deposited at some point in the body. As a result, different parts of the body, such as the skin or joints, may become sick with lupus or get inflamed.

In lupus, if a part of the body is affected, it will become hot, red, swollen, and sometimes tender. Painful swollen joints (showing the existence of arthritis); reddened skin (indicating a rash); hair loss (indicating alopecia); hands changing color in the cold (pointing to Raynaud's phenomenon); and mouth sores are all symptoms of the disease. In spite of the discomfort and pain these symptoms cause, they do not bring serious harm to the body's functions and can be treated by medications. In children and adolescents, lupus could affect the internal organs, making the problem more serious.

If the kidneys become inflamed in children, this could develop into nephritis. For those whose brain is affected, they may have seizures, serious mood changes, or hallucinations. In others, kidneys affected by lupus could mean fluid around the heart or lungs. It is clearly important to prevent internal organs from being affected by lupus. To achieve that, regular visits to the doctor for evaluations such as blood and urine tests are mandatory.

In the early stage when only blood tests show an abnormality, treatment for lupus is much easier than later, when one or more organs has become inflamed, requiring more medications. Most children and adolescents get the warning signs early through blood tests, making early treatment possible.

Clinical Manifestations

Renal
In a randomly selected group of lupus patients, 30%–50% may exhibit urine and kidney abnormalities. However, 80% of children and 60% of adults may subsequently develop overt kidney disease. Development of nephritis in patients who developed lupus after the age of fifty years is very uncommon, with less than 5% being affected.

All lupus patients with kidney disease tend to lose protein in the urine, with a significant number of them showing microscopic hematuria, which means blood loss in the urine. These patients also have decreased kidney function, and many may lose kidney function rapidly. Hypertension is not more prevalent in lupus patients with kidney inflammation, but it is more common in those with severe lupus. Bladder involvement is also prominent. However, in cases of early recognition and management of SLE, end-stage renal disease develops in fewer than 5% of patients.

Extrarenal
SLE is a disease known as "the great imitator" because it often mimics or is mistaken for other disorders. The symptoms of SLE vary considerably, and appear and disappear unpredictably. Diagnosis can be confusing. Some people suffer unexplained facets of this disorder for years without treatment.

Common initial symptoms include fever, malaise, fatigue, muscle pain, and temporary loss of cognitive function. Other features emerge as manifestations of the body organs when involved.

Though 65% of those with lupus may develop skin disease at some point or other, 30% will have skin involvement, and of these, 30% to 50% exhibit the typical butterfly rash on the face. Some develop red scaly patches on the skin. Hair loss, and mouth, nasal, and vaginal ulcers, may also be observed in these patients.

Patients commonly seek medical attention for joint pain. All joints may be affected, but the small joints of the hands and wrist are usually affected. It is believed that more than 90% of lupus patients develop joint and/or muscle pain at some point during the course of this disorder. Lupus arthritis is generally less disabling than osteoarthritis or rheumatoid arthritis and does not lead to destructive arthropathy. However, SLE is associated with an increased risk of bone fractures in relatively young women.

Anemia and iron deficiency may develop in greater than 50% of cases. Low platelets and white blood cell counts may result from lupus itself or from the drugs used to treat lupus.

Lupus patients may experience inflammation of the heart covering, heart muscle, and heart valves. Usually the mitral valve and tricuspid valves are affected, and involvement is characteristically noninfective. Atherosclerosis is often present and progresses rapidly in lupus patients as compared to the general population.

The involvement of the lungs includes inflammation of the lung covering (pleura), fluid accumulation in the pleural cavity, lupus pneumonitis, chronic interstitial disease, pulmonary hypertension, pulmonary embolism, pulmonary hemorrhage, and shrinking lung disease.

Lupus can affect both the central and the peripheral nervous system. The diagnosis of neuropsychiatric involvement in this disorder presents a great challenge in medicine, as it may exhibit many patterns of symptoms, some of which may mimic an infectious process or stroke. The most common symptom is headache. Other manifestations include cognitive dysfunction, seizures, anxiety and mood disorders, cerebrovascular disease, polyneuropathy, and psychosis. Intracranial pressure may increase with attendant complications. Many other neuropsychiatric complications are rarely observed in SLE.

Treatment

The treatment of SLE involves preventing flare-ups and reducing their severity and duration when present. Treatment includes corticosteroids and antimalarial drugs. Renal involvement requires different cytotoxic drugs depending on the histologic changes, the severity of disease, and renal function.

Sunlight is known to exacerbate the disease and should be avoided. Occupational exposure to silica, pesticides, and mercury may also make the disease worse.

Transplantation

There may be conflicting results. Generally, there is no difference in graft survival and patient mortality compared to nonlupus transplant recipients after the first cadaveric and living-related kidney transplant. The reported rates of recurrence are also widely variable; however, recurrence with graft failure occurs at a rate comparable to that of all allograft transplants and accounts for less than 4%.

Spread of Lupus by Population

Today, the rate of lupus varies among countries, and is influenced by ethnicity and gender. As far as the rise in its incidence, it is unclear if it can be attributed to better diagnosis or to increasing frequency of the disease.

In the United States, the prevalence of SLE is estimated at 53 per 100,000, translating to about 159,000 out of more than 300 million people, while in Northern Europe it has captured the lives of almost 40 out of every 100,000 individuals. The rate is much higher in people of Afro-Caribbean descent and reaches as high as 159 per 100,000.

Comparing the disease's behavior among African Americans and Caucasians, it has been observed that the former have a threefold increased incidence of lupus, as they develop the disease at a younger age, with earlier setting in of nephritis and with higher mortality rate. There is a tendency of SLE to impact more lives and with far greater severity in people of non-European descent. This is true also for Hispanics and Asians, who also face severe nephritis compared to Americans. Recent studies show a higher proportion of lupus patients receiving dialytic therapy for chronic kidney disease. The mortality outcome in lupus patients receiving dialysis is not different from that of the overall dialysis patient population.

Like many autoimmune diseases, lupus is primarily a disease affecting young women, with the incidence at its peak between the ages of fifteen and forty years. However, it can be found among people of all ages, infants to people of advanced ages. The female-to-male ratio rises from 2:1 in prepubescent children, up to 4.5:1 in adolescents, to 8:1 in adults, and decreases to 2:1 in patients over sixty years of age. While the estrogen hormone in females seems to be a precipitating factor in the emergence of lupus, in males the hormone androgen plays a protective role, so much so that lupus does not favor the male gender.

Another interesting aspect of lupus is that it appears to display familial aggregation, with higher prevalence among first-degree relatives. In monozygotic twins, SLE occurs concordantly in as high as 25% to 50%, while only 5% of dizygotic twins share the condition. In extended families, this disease may be associated with other autoimmune disorders, such as hemolytic anemia, thyroiditis, and idiopathic thrombocytopenia purpura. However, most cases of SLE are sporadic.

CKD MANAGEMENT, ISSUES, AND TREATMENTS

Dr. Mohammad Akmal

Hyperparathyroidism

Hyperparathyroidism is a common complication of chronic kidney disease. The increase in parathyroid hormone generally follows the decline in kidney function. Parathyroid glands regulate calcium levels in the blood, and hyperparathyroidism is caused by improper calcium regulation. Four pairs of parathyroid glands are situated behind the thyroid gland to monitor and control calcium in the blood and bones by secreting parathyroid hormone (PTH).

Hyperparathyroidism occurs when one or more parathyroid glands enlarge or develop into a tumor and subsequently releases large quantities of parathyroid hormone into the blood. Excess parathyroid hormone goes through the blood into bones and activates cells in the bone that eat away the bone. Then multiple complications associated with excess parathyroid hormone develop. Dietary phosphorous restriction, vitamin D, vitamin-like agents, and specific therapy may arrest or reverse this condition. In some cases surgical removal of two-thirds of the glands may be needed.

Hyperphosphatemia (high levels of phosphorous) is common particularly in late stages of chronic kidney disease (CKD). As CKD advances, phosphorous regulation declines and loss of phosphorous via the kidney occurs, at which point hyperphosphatemia develops. Observational studies have determined that hyperphosphatemia is an independent cardiovascular risk factor in CKD. Mechanistically, it has been suggested that it directly stimulates vascular calcification. Cardiovascular calcification contributes to extreme mortality in CKD. Dietary restrictions and phosphate binders are used to control phosphorus levels in the blood.

Problems Created by Excess Phosphorus, Excess Calcium, and Heightened Levels of Parathyroid Hormone

The blood level of parathyroid hormone plays a critical role in controlling calcium and phosphorous levels. This complex complication results from many factors. High phosphorous plays a pivotal role in inducing hyperparathyroidism. The multiple complications may affect organs such as the brain and the skin, and other body parts of the body like the bones and blood cells.

In the case of a patient we'll call "Lucy," hyperparathyroidism caused the following:

- enlarged heart with poor function
- very high phosphorous and calcium levels, meaning that calcium deposition in tissues and bone abnormalities developed
- large ball-like abnormalities in both shoulders

The combination of her conditions made parathyroidectomy inevitable. Three and one-half of her parathyroid glands were removed.

The next step was to resolve calcium deposition around her shoulders.

Hyperparathyroidism begins to develop when kidney function is about 60% and is almost a universal finding in dialysis patients. It is associated with damage to many tissues and organs in the body in dialysis patients. As the kidney fails significantly, there is reduced production of active vitamin D by the kidney and development of hyperphosphatemia. To simplify, these factors directly stimulate the production of parathyroid hormone and also indirectly cause a reduction in blood calcium. Hyperphosphatemia, in addition to many complications of CKD, also contributes to cardiovascular disease.

Tuberculosis

TB peritonitis is uncommon, but unusual features like night sweats, weight loss, and unexplained fevers should be attended to, particularly in peritoneal dialysis patients from countries with TB endemics and patients with poor immune systems, as with AIDS.

Hepatitis C

Overall, the global incidence of hepatitis C is 3.3%. Long-term infection with hepatitis C (HCV), known as chronic hepatitis C, is usually a silent for decades, until the liver is significantly damaged by the virus, resulting in signs and symptoms of liver disease. Chronic hepatitis begins with an acute phase, which usually goes undetected as it rarely leads to symptoms. If symptoms develop, they may include jaundice, nausea, fever, and muscle aches. The acute phase appears one to three months after exposure to the virus and lasts two weeks to three months. The acute phase may not become chronic. In about 14%–50% of cases, there is spontaneous viral clearance, and HCV is also responsive to antiviral therapy.

The infection spreads when contaminated blood enters the blood of a person. Worldwide, HCV exists in several forms known as genotypes. Type 1 is more common in North America and Europe, where the presence of type 2 is less common. These two types are found throughout the world. However, other genotypes cause infection in the majority of patients in the Middle East, Asia, and Africa. Even though chronic hepatitis C runs a similar course regardless of the genotype, treatment varies depending on genotype.

Risk factors for HCV are as follows:

1. A health care worker exposed to infected blood, which could occur if the skin is pierced by an infected needle
2. Injected or inhaled illicit drugs
3. Persons with HIV infection
4. Tattoo or piercing with an unsterile equipment
5. Blood transfusion or organ transplantation before 1992
6. Transfusion of clotting factor concentrates before 1987
7. Long-term hemodialytic therapy
8. Infant born to a hepatitis C–infected woman
9. History of ever being in prison

The highest incidence is in people born between 1945 and 1965.

Complications
After twenty to thirty years of infection with hepatitis C, liver cirrhosis and advanced liver failure may occur. Liver cancer may develop in a small number of cases. Hepatitis C is also associated with many extrahepatic manifestations, including impaired glucose metabolism, cryoglobulinemic vasculitis, B-cell non-Hodgkin lymphoma, and chronic kidney disease. Membranous and membranoproliferative glomerulonephritis, and cryoglobulinemia-induced vasculitis, are other significant associated medical conditions.

Diagnosis and treatment
Hepatitis C is diagnosed with a special MRI, special ultrasound, and biopsy. Antiviral treatment used at appropriate times is very effective. Transplantation in appropriate cases is also offered.

Hepatitis B
The incidence of this disease is highest in the Western Pacific Region and Africa, with more than 6% of the adult population being affected. The prevalence in the eastern Mediterranean region is 3.3%; in Southeast Asia, 2.0%; in the European region, 1.6%; and in the Americas, 0.7%.

The renal diseases most commonly associated with hepatitis B (HBV) infection include membranous nephropathy, membranoproliferative glomerulonephritis and polyarteritis nodosa. Hepatitis B can also cause cirrhosis of liver, liver failure, and cancer.

It spreads when people come in contact with the blood, open sores, or body fluid of someone with the hepatitis B virus. In most cases, the disease does not last a long time, as the body fights off the infection within a few months and the person becomes immune for the rest of his or her life.

Some people fail to get rid of the infection. If it lasts for more than six months, they become carriers, even if they are symptom-free, and are able to transmit the disease to others.

Diagnosis
Diagnosis is made with a blood test for the hepatitis B virus, and with liver biopsy if the disease becomes chronic.

Treatment
If the patient is exposed to the virus, within two weeks consult a doctor, who will give a vaccine and hepatitis B immunoglobulin, which will help the immune system fight off the infection. The patient will be advised against alcohol consumption and acetaminophen ingestion. Early recognition and appropriate antiviral therapy may reduce liver cirrhosis, liver failure, and cancer.

Multiple Myeloma
Multiple myeloma was known to the world as early as 1844, when Samuel Solly reported a well-documented case. A few years later, a London trader, Alexander McBean, was found to be excreting a large amount of protein. In 1847 Henry Bence Jones, a physician and chemist, identified a globulin protein, suggesting it as multiple myeloma. Thereafter this protein was referred to by his name.

Magnesium

Magnesium is as an essential metal needed in many functions of the human cells. The kidney plays a very important role in magnesium metabolism. Magnesium is the second-most abundant intracellular cation and, overall, the fourth-most abundant cation. It plays a fundamental role in many functions of the cell, including energy transfer and storage; protein, carbohydrate, and fat metabolism; maintenance of normal cell membrane function; and regulation of parathyroid hormone (PTH) secretion. Systemically, magnesium lowers blood pressure and alters peripheral vascular resistance. It is a naturally occurring crystal inhibitor and plays a role in preventing kidney stones.

The average body content of magnesium is 25 grams, and 60% is found in bone, 20% in muscle, and the remaining 20% in soft tissue and the liver. About 99% of total body magnesium is in the cells and is bone dependent, and 1% is outside the cells.

In advanced chronic kidney disease, blood levels of magnesium are increased. On the other hand, low levels of magnesium may result in insulin resistance, diabetes, hypertension, atherosclerosis, and inflammation. These factors play a major role in the progression of chronic kidney disease. Moreover, a low level of magnesium has been associated with cardiovascular disease and all-cause mortality in end-stage renal disease (also known as chronic kidney disease, or CKD). Low magnesium levels may also lead to a decline in kidney function in CKD and to poor function and survival of the kidneys in kidney transplant patients. How low a magnesium level causes these abnormalities is not known. Further studies are needed in chronic kidney disease and dialysis patients for clarification. However, studies suggest that high magnesium levels and magnesium supplementation may reduce vascular calcification in CKD.

Abnormalities of magnesium levels, such as hypomagnesemia (low blood levels of magnesium), can result in disturbances in nearly every organ system and can cause potentially fatal complications (e.g., arrhythmia, coronary artery vasospasm, hypertension, coronary artery disease, nerve and muscle damage, osteoporosis, diabetes, and kidney stones). These abnormalities are also associated with many other miscellaneous conditions (e.g., migraine, asthma, chronic fatigue syndrome, sudden death in athletes, and sudden infant death syndrome) secondary to this poorly understood mechanism.

Despite the well-recognized importance of magnesium, low and high levels have been documented in ill patients, as a result of which magnesium has occasionally been called the "forgotten cation."

The factors that control magnesium metabolism are absorption from the gut and loss in the urine. The average American diet contains about 360 mg of magnesium daily. Magnesium is abundantly found in green vegetables, cereals, grains, nuts, legumes, and chocolate. Vegetables, meats, fish, and fruits contain intermediate quantities. Magnesium content is severely decreased by cooking and food processing, and thus a large segment of the population consume less than the required allowance.

Magnesium is principally absorbed in the small intestine. In normal circumstances, 30%–40% of the magnesium is absorbed. Under conditions of low magnesium intake, a higher percentage is absorbed depending on the amount of magnesium ingested.

The rate of risk of hypomagnesemia can be summarized as follows:

- 2% in the general population
- 10%–20% in hospitalized patients
- 50%–60% in intensive care unit (ICU) patients
- 30%–80% in persons with alcoholism
- 25% in outpatients with diabetes

One reason oxalate is not usually readily absorbed from the gut is that it is complexed with calcium to a large degree. Ordinarily, little fat reaches the colon. However, in fat malabsorptive states, fatty acids reach the colon and bind calcium, thus freeing up oxalate for absorption. Bile acid malabsorption might also contribute by inuring intestinal cells and increasing colonic permeability. Common causes of enteric hyperoxaluria include the now jejunoileal bypass, modern bariatric procedures, inflammatory disease like Crohn's disease, and intestinal resection.

Hemodialysis

For millions of the patients with end-stage renal disease (ESRD) worldwide, hemodialysis has become a routine therapy. This lifesaving therapy has been applied for more than forty years. The most common cause of end-stage renal disease is diabetes, followed by hypertension.

The highest prevalence rate for ESRD is found in Japan, at 2,045 per million, followed by the United States, with a rate of 1,509 per million. Fifty-two percent of the global dialysis population resides in Japan, the United States, Germany, and Brazil, which together make up 11% of the world population.

There is a recurrent controversy involving the question of whether peritoneal dialysis (PD) or hemodialysis (HD) is the superior therapy. This is a difficult question to answer with certainty because selection for the two treatments is biased and not random. In general, patients selected for PD have fewer comorbid conditions independent of other factors that may influence modality selection.

Among the accepted criteria for initiating dialysis are creatinine clearance of 15 ml/min for diabetics and 10 L/min for nondiabetics.

The following factors improve the morbidity and mortality rates: adherence to the prescribed dietary and fluid restrictions; control of blood pressure (BP); appropriate correction of anemia; control of calcium, phosphorus, and hyperparathyroidism; control of hyperlipidemia; cardiovascular monitoring; adequacy of dialysis; control of diabetes in diabetics; and prevention of infection and intradialytic hypotension.

Hypotension

It is the most common acute complication of HD, occurring in approximately 20%–50% of the dialytic treatments. A greater number of episodes are encountered in older patients and women. A drop in BP during dialysis treatment, especially when it occurs frequently, is associated with an increased rate of morbidity and mortality. The dialysis procedure is considered to be made up of two separable procedures, convection and diffusion.

Convection refers to the movement of fluid and solute brought by pressure across the dialysis membrane (transmembrane pressure). The higher the transmembrane pressure, the greater the movement of fluid and solute across the dialysis membrane.

The process of fluid removal by the hydraulic force is termed ultrafiltration (UF). During isolated UF, a progressive increase in total systemic vascular resistance maintains BP as fluid is removed. When diffusion is added to UF (usual dialysis treatment, combination of UF and diffusion), thermal energy can be transferred from heated dialysis to the patient, resulting in vasodilatation and increased flow to the skin. As a result, vasoconstriction becomes less effective, and maintenance of central blood volume may be impaired when fluid is removed. Cardiac output and BP are maintained by heart rate and, in some instances, by an increase in myocardial contractility. Unfortunately, when intravascular volume is low, the two aforementioned factors may fail to maintain a tolerable BP. Furthermore, significant heart disease in dialysis patients often limits the ability of the heart and the blood vessels to appropriately respond to the stress of fluid removal. Impaired autonomic function in these patients also limits the reflex vasoconstriction response during hypotensive episodes.

A very large intradialytic weight gain cannot be easily removed during a typical treatment period (3.5 to 4 hours), even in the presence of fluid overload, as refilling of intravascular space is time dependent. Hypotension in these patients is an exponential function of the rate of fluid removal, especially if removed in excess of 1.5 L/hr. Hypotension can occur in dialysis patients who are at or below estimated dry weight when volume shifts no longer are able to compensate for intravascular depletion and maintain BP. Estimated dry weight is defined as the weight below which the patient develops symptomatic hypotension in the absence of edema and excessive weight gain during dialysis.

Other factors that may contribute to hypotension include antihypertensive medications, low hematocrit, arrhythmia, poor cardiac function, pericardial effusion, sepsis, and inappropriately large size of the dialyzer.

Management

The first step is to determine whether the hypotension occurs early or late in the dialysis treatment. If it occurs late in the treatment in a patient who was previously stable and free from edema and heart failure, the likely cause will be underestimated dry weight. Therefore, reducing the UF during dialysis, and effectively raising dry weight after dialysis, will correct the hypotension. In contrast, the patient who gains an excessive amount of weight between dialysis treatments may become hypotensive early in treatment before dry weight is achieved because the rate at which fluid can be mobilized to refill the intravascular space is limited. These patients are required to limit excessive weight gain between dialysis treatments and increase the frequency and duration of treatment. Specific management of the aforementioned factors will also be needed.

Hypotension, when it occurs, is treated by placing the patient in the Trendelenburg position, administering 100–200 ml normal saline bolus, and reducing UF, at least temporarily. Other alternative treatments are with mannitol, glucose, hypertonic saline, and albumin. In some individuals, supplemental oxygen may be useful to improve hypoxemia and cardiac contractility.

Infection

Infection, the second leading cause of death in HD patients, is responsible for a mortality rate of 12%–22%. Septicemia accounts for 75% of these infections. Overall, the annual percentage of mortality resulting from sepsis is one hundredfold to three hundredfold higher than in the general population. Dialysis access is an important risk factor, and using a catheter presents a much higher sepsis risk compared to using dialysis access.

Fever in the dialysis patient should alert the physician to the strong possibility of infection.

Muscle Cramps

Muscle cramps are the second most common reported complication of HD, occurring in as many as 20% of dialysis treatments. The pathogenesis remains uncertain but appears to be higher when UF rates are high during hypotension in dialysis, and when dialysate with low sodium concentration is employed, indicating development of cramps caused by extracellular volume contraction.

Reducing UF rates, IV normal saline (200 ml), or a solution of 50% dextrose in water, 5 ml, may help. The pain from severe cramps may be alleviated by administration of diazepam, but this carries with it the risk of hypotension.

Quinine sulfate is effective in preventing cramps if administered one to two hours before dialysis. It increases the refractory period and excitability of skeletal muscles. Monitor for development of thrombocytopenia. Vitamin E and carnitine have also been tried, with variable effects.

Peritoneal Dialysis

In Germany in the 1920s, Georg Ganter was the first person to perform peritoneal dialysis (PD). Russell Palmer developed a catheter made of silicon rubber and used it to treat small number of patients with acute renal failure in the 1940s. The process for dialysis continued to improve, and first began to be utilized in patients with chronic end-stage renal failure. Subsequently, pioneers like Henry Tenckhoff developed cuffed catheters and automated cycling equipment. Intermittent PD to treat end-stage renal disease had become relatively more common by the mid-1970s. Subsequently, it evolved into a modality utilized to treat thousands of patients after the development of continuous ambulatory peritoneal dialysis (CAPD) by Jack Moncrief and Robert Popovich in 1977. With the passage of time, Dimitrios Oreopoulos and Karl Nolph, along with their colleagues, made further modifications that have facilitated the widespread use of CAPD. The low cost, the relatively simple technique, and the ease with which it can be used at home by the patient has made CAPD a popular dialysis modality.

PD has seen enormous success for over thirty years, which has been made possible by better understanding of human anatomy and physiology—essential for this modality and recognition of complications.

Peritonitis

This is a leading cause of complication, resulting in increased morbidity, technique failure, hospitalizations, and occasionally mortality. Its frequency has decreased over the years because of more awareness, early recognition, improved technique, and better preventive measures. It can be caused by gram positive organisms, gram negative organisms, fungi, and antitubercular treatment.

Diagnosis

Three cardinal features of peritonitis are cloudy effluent, abdominal pain, and a positive effluent culture. Typically, these three are present. However, two of three features are sufficient to make a convincing diagnosis.

- A patient with PD presenting with cloudy effluent is likely to have peritonitis, unless proven otherwise.
- Abdominal pain may precede cloudy effluent, and intensity of pain varies with the type of organism causing the infection.
- With pseudomonas and fungal peritonitis, pain is generally more severe.
- The presence of high fever is not typical of PD peritonitis and indicates sepsis.
- Effluent should be sent for total and differential white blood count (WBC), gram stain, and blood culture before antibiotic therapy is initiated.
- Effluent WBC > 100 cells/l, along with neutrophils > 50%, are suggestive of peritonitis. With proper culture technique, effluent should be positive in 80%–90% of peritonitis cases.
- A negative culture with effluent leukocytosis and suggestive symptoms of peritonitis may indicate fastidious organisms, preexisting antibiotic therapy, inadequate collection and sample technique, nonbacterial infection, or laboratory problems. Repeat culture may become positive. With widespread use of antibiotics, infection secondary to resistant organisms has become more prevalent.

Management

The important considerations are the initial choice of empiric antibiotic therapy prior to identification of organisms, subsequent choice, and duration of therapy depending on culture results. Another important question is when and whether to remove the PD catheter from people with severe infections.

Renal Transplantation

Renal transplantation is the treatment of choice for end-stage renal disease (ESRD), but unfortunately for a small number of patients, as most of these patients are never evaluated for transplantation. In the USA, the five-year dialysis mortality rate is 70%.

Renal transplantation has shown significant improvement in early graft survival and long-term graft function, making it a more cost-effective alternative to dialysis. The transplantation activity in developing countries is poor, with a rate of less than 10 per million population (pmp), in contrast to that in developed countries, at 45 to 50 pmp. With an estimated world incidence of end-stage renal disease of 80–110 pmp, developed countries fulfill 30%–35% of their needs, in contrast to 1%–2% of developing countries. It has progressed from the first kidney transplantation in identical twins in Boston in 1951 to more than 447,000 to date.

Before immunosuppression was available, renal transplantation was limited to identical twins and the majority of the patients with ESRD could not receive transplantation. Since the introduction of immunosuppressive therapy, and with continuing improvement in such therapy and effective newer agents, there has been a significant impact on both patients and graft survival. Currently, the patient's one-year graft survival rate exceeds 90% in most transplant centers in the USA.

Although approximately only 25% of adult patients on dialysis and perhaps 95% of pediatric patients with ESRD are referred for transplantation evaluation, the waiting list for kidney transplantation has grown very large.

With increasing interest in living donation, and possibly with of the introduction of laparoscopic donor nephrectomy in 1994, has come not only a substantial growth in living-donor transplants but also shorter waiting times for kidneys and improved outcomes of transplants.

Some conditions are known to recur in the transplanted kidney (e.g., IgA nephropathy, oxalises, certain types of glomerular disease, and diabetes). However, the rate of recurrence is low enough to justify transplantation.

There are a number of contraindications for renal transplantation, some for surgery, others for immunosuppression, and still others derived from various concomitant disorders.

Contraindications for surgery include metastatic cancer, hepatic insufficiency (people who suffer with this may be candidates for liver and kidney transplantation), severe cardiac and peripheral vascular disease, serious conditions that are unlikely to improve after renal transplantation, repeated episodes of medical noncompliance, and inability to perform rehabilitation adequately after transplantation.

HIV with a positive blood test is not a contraindication for kidney transplantation provided that the patient has a CD4 count greater than 200/L for at least six months and undetectable HIV RNA, is without any major infections or neoplastic complications, and has been stable on antiretroviral therapy for at least three months. Adverse effects of immunosuppressive drugs may exacerbate atherosclerosis, hypertension, diabetes, and lipid disorders and therefore increase cardiac risk after transplantation. Cardiac disease is the most common cause of death in these patients.

Contraindications for immunosuppression are infection and malignancy. Acute infection should be fully resolved at the time of transplantation. In general, one should wait for about five years after successful treatment of breast cancer, colorectal cancer, melanoma, diffuse bladder cancer, and non-in-situ ovarian cancer. The risk of recurrence is about 50% if the transplant is performed within two years of such treatment, about 35% if it is performed between two and five years, and about only 10% if it is done after five years.

Some tumors may allow shorter waiting list (e.g., nodules of prostatic cancer and focal bladder carcinoma; one year (or even less) is reasonable for in situ uterine carcinoma and some renal tumors, including 9 clear cell, Wilms, and urothelioma; and for basal cell skin carcinoma, no waiting time at all may be reasonable.

The prognosis after kidney transplantation is generally excellent, with one-year graft survival rates ranging from 90% to 95%. HLA-identical transplants from living related donors have the best graft survival rate, whereas transplant from complete mismatch cadaveric donors have the worst.

Post-transplant infections are a major problem in developing countries, with 15% of transplant patients developing tuberculosis, 30% cytomegalic problems, and nearly 50% bacterial infection.

(Any reference made in the foregoing pages is only indicative. Please get your medications prescribed through your doctor. Your doctor knows your health better. The above guidance is for you to understand how some issues you could encounter may be handled.)

SAFE PREGNANCY FOR THE PATIENT AND THE UNBORN

Dr. Mohammad Akmal

If a patient with chronic kidney disease gets pregnant, it puts both mother and unborn child at high risk. Before conception, a patient should discuss the possibility of conception, so physicians can ensure that medications for kidney disease that could have an adverse effect on pregnancy and place the mother and the fetus at risk are not administered. Appropriate birth control medications for women of childbearing age should be advised.

Patients with chronic kidney disease (stages 1 and 2), with normal blood pressure and with little or no protein in the urine, may have a normal pregnancy.

For patients with moderate to severe chronic disease (stages 3–5), the risk of complication is much greater. They need close monitoring during pregnancy.

Pregnancy during dialysis (peritoneal or hemodialysis) is an uncommon event. The risks to mother and fetus are significantly higher. More frequent dialysis; blood pressure, fluids, and electrolytes monitoring; and anemia correction are important aspects for a safe delivery. With such measures, normal pregnancies have been reported.

Pregnancy in kidney transplant patients should be contemplated only by patients who have a functioning kidney transplant, stable kidney function and blood pressure, and good medical and psychologic condition for more than one year—and after detailed discussion with their nephrologist. Certain drugs that will affect kidney function and may have detrimental effects on the fetus must be avoided.

PATIENT-CENTRIC ASPECTS: TRAUMA AND THE NEED FOR SUPPORT

Vasundhara Raghavan

Early Challenges of Kidney Disease

I recall the first time we left the nephrologist's clinic and were driving home. All of us were quiet—different people thinking about different aspects. My son was fifteen and a half years old. He had his own teenage worries. As a mother I was overwhelmed and hence unsure how to tackle such a sensitive subject. It was far easier to remain quiet. But my husband, being a practical person with a scientific mind, used the ride to seek answers. He made a logical assessment of the situation.

Later, at home, he took the discussions to a different level. It began with making an assessment of our son's sad state, emphasizing problems likely to be encountered. And all the dangers were laid threadbare, enough to make my stomach churn with fear.

All negative aspects of the disease and dangers exposed, he talked about an alternative way of approaching the subject: how to turn the negatives into positives! Even as these evaluations were happening, like a mother hen I floated around the house as if I were all-pervasive. The truth is, I was worried that the teenager was getting too much information that would terrify him!

But I was wrong.

It worked wonderfully. This was a big lesson I learned about life. Terror exposes a reason to fight for life. Some people roll up their sleeves and get to work, whereas others may hide under the couch.

In life, we need to make a choice. We need to walk onto the battlefield and face the adversary—an eye for eye. What transpired in our household that day and a few days thereafter gave us the courage to go all out to explode the myth that there's no chance for survival!

The value of logical thinking will be evident in a short while.

Making a Plan to Handle the Diagnosis and Manage the Disease

Any patient leaving a kidney specialist's room comes out in a state of shock.

If others accompany the person, their reactions are similar. From that moment, subconsciously a certain clock begins ticking inside them spelling death. Irrespective of the person's age and vocation, the patient makes the easy choice:

- to drown in self-pity and stop all activity
- to believe his or her existence is under threat (of course, it is, but this needs to be downplayed!)

- to wonder about the value of education or staying employed
- to focus only on health care

During the early days kidney patients had no capacity to plan and determine their future quality of life. For a mind lost in the woods, gone is the capacity to notice the brightness and warmth of the sun, wonder about the clear blue sky, hear the chirping of the birds, or see the brilliance of the silver stars in the dark of the night. These are nature's elements that could otherwise guide them to safety.

Kidney patients need *someone* at that early stage to show compassion with an understanding nod or a gentle touch, which generates a feeling of dependability. Over time a conversation could build a rapport and draw the kidney patient toward the right approach. Someone needs show the kidney patient that contemplating any drastic action should actually be placed right at the bottom of their checklist.

Placed up front as a *priority* should be the following things:

- first, securing one's fort from all dangers, including being driven by one's own erratic mind.
- making a plan for survival

Our decision-making process went something like this:

1. We spent a few hours trying to understand what had happened. What had we done wrong that landed us in this situation?
2. We found out as much about the disease as possible.
3. We came to an understanding of the current stage of the disease and assessed how much time might be locked up before reaching next stage. Or, if we had such power, to assess if there was any safe period at all.
4. Asking questions such as, What is dialysis? What are the types available? How many people survive kidney disease? This topic is painful, as death stares you straight in the eye.
5. Asking other questions, such as, How can we get a transplant? What is the success rate? Who is medically eligible? What are the transplant laws?
6. And yes, importantly we considered the diet!
7. We determined our finances: Where would funds come for this treatment?

All the skeletons were now out of the closet. Upon inspecting things closely to understand all aspects completely, we were drowned in worry, as each facet looked scarier than the earlier one.

Though no. 7 is finances, placed in the last slot as if to say, *Money cannot buy everything,* in the case of chronic kidney disease it ranks *first.* Every kidney patient who doesn't have this commodity feels stranded in the middle of a huge deluge. Every rich patient believes they can fight chronic kidney disease (CKD) with this powerful weapon, only to realize that indeed money cannot buy everything! Money, money, and more money is needed to get treated and continue living.

Logical thinking can help you confront your fears and control them. Logic is the guide that leads you to a clear thinking zone. Death is in the cards for everyone; life is there for people who want to survive and in whom stirs the *will* to do so. The will to survive is very dim, but it gathers momentum as you reach each roadblock. You have to tell yourself that it is a delusion and that such roadblocks can be surmounted. You need to plan how to leap forward.

Let's get back to my family's way of handling kidney disease.

Over the next few weeks, we collected information. My husband made it like a classroom where both my sons were actively participating. I was in hiding. (As a mother, my sense of guilt was at its height.) Emotional outbursts were intermittent, and my son, who was an exuberant and promising young lad, was now spending more time by himself. At odd times he was found surfing the internet for the latest information.

But we made a plan that we followed through on, with many modifications. At the top of the list was the unspoken and spoken agenda: to complete schooling, graduate, and be on a career path so the future would present a smoother road moving in some direction.

Research tells us that a person who continues to be employed is happier.

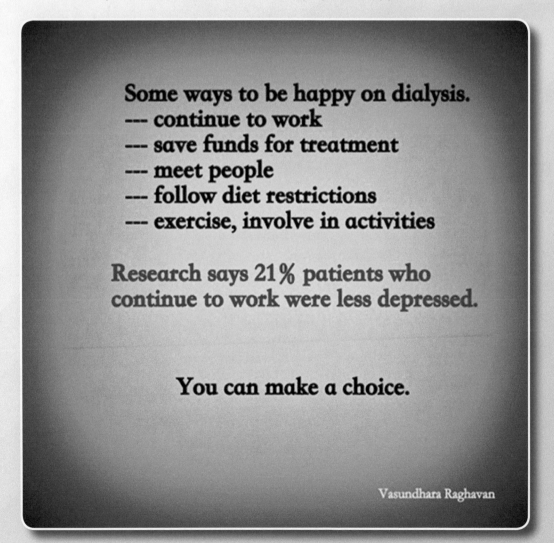

Some ways to be happy on dialysis.
--- **continue to work**
--- **save funds for treatment**
--- **meet people**
--- **follow diet restrictions**
--- **exercise, involve in activities**

Research says 21% patients who continue to work were less depressed.

You can make a choice.

Vasundhara Raghavan

The foregoing graphic presents a sample plan. Make your own survival plan. It can be as exotic as you want it to be, but follow your heart and map your journey so that you can live with all your mental capacities intact.

Airtight plans fail, as we are never sure of the obstacles ahead. Nevertheless, it is important to break down all the walls and try to penetrate them. Also, never let your fear build its own hillock!

Every person has his or her own individual mental process for handling a serious disease. It is important to make your own plan.

Find an Outlet for Your Emotions

An emotional outburst is a statement of the person's mental state. Let me say it here and now: It is very much allowed! Go do it.

It is totally permitted to feel the earth slip from beneath your feet, to feel ruined and that life is at its natural end. There's no need to say "I love life" and live with false confidence. That could shatter the first time you face resistance.

It's almost as if you are in a tunnel and a huge rock was blocking the end so no light could penetrate. You have a choice to sit and quietly work on the rock. Your own patience and persistence will never go unnoticed. Slowly, chips of the rock will fall at your feet when you hit it, apply pressure. When you're frustrated, rest. Give vent to your feelings. But go back to doing the only thing possible: breaking the barrier.

The world respects a person who tries hard. People are amazing when it comes to putting you on a pedestal and worshipping you for your perseverance. Work gets recognized. Courage gets rewarded.

Imagine the total helplessness of a beggar who has only a worn-out shirt with his pockets empty and with hunger gnawing him. He can't see any reason to live. It's like he can see no future at all.

That empty feeling is just what chronic kidney disease awakens in you. You feel cheated as if robbed of something precious. So please feel free to express yourself and yell at the world around you. But after that, calm your nerves. Work on making a resolution to survive.

On Facebook, my social media friend Mark Rosen has a special group. We interacted a little to understand each person's first reaction to chronic kidney disease. Such a great revelation! So many stood tall amid the sands of time, weathering bruises of ego and of body, and yet had made it through to share their testimonies with others.

Some heart-wrenching observations from Facebook are listed below.

Joan Gregory said, "Shock, some hopelessness and some dread. That was ten years ago. I've stayed around the same numbers since then (stage 3b). Still it's worrisome!"

Virginia Halsey remarked, "Charles and I were both scared to death of what would come next!"

Gail Rae-Garwood made a big statement: "Terror, abject terror! I thought I was being given a death sentence. Boy, was I ever wrong!"

Dee Moore's speculation tells us how many people could save their kidney: "I didn't really think much about it. It happened some twenty years ago. I didn't feel bad. There was no symptom, but there was protein in the urine. I knew nothing about creatinine at that time. But today I'm on dialysis. I wonder, if I had thought a little bit more about it, met a doctor, would it have been a different situation?"

Patty Powell Oxley's fear was very real. "As a newly retired acute care RN, I was scared and felt hopeless. I knew about kidney disease!"

Magda Bonacina's confession speaks volumes: "For me: fear … also because [my] nephrologists didn't explain much!

Mare Daly talks of her husband: "Worried and immediately researched to find the best nephrologist in [New Jersey] and made an appointment for my husband. He's doing great now; battled CKD eighteen years, did PD for two years, and is now six months post-transplant from our son. Life is wonderful again. Positiveness and not letting this disease define you is key! 🩶🖤

Mark Rosen, formidable as he is, said simply, "Fear."

Jim Bishop told us a lot: "The kidney disease was diagnosed during a string of heart attacks that led to open heart surgery. I believe the initial reaction was one of being irritated by one more complication."

Lyn Adams Hanlon said, "I was pissed off with my primary doctor. He knew my numbers and said nothing so that I don't worry till I was well into third stage already. Why do they not tell me? It could have been addressed then, before it got so far into fourth stage with a GFR of 28."

Sherry Simons told us about dreams: "For me it was fear. I thought, *I have so much that I still want to do!* But I've realized life is a blessing. I will not give in to my deep fears. Yes, it's hard, but live each day thankful!"

From all this, clearly we have something to work on.

1. Talk to your doctor. Get your doubts cleared. Your health is your concern. Doctors have many patients and are busy with other serious cases. You have only your case to deal with. Maintain a good rapport with your doctor. While discussing, be a good listener. You will learn many useful things.
2. Talk to your family and friends about your illness. Your sharing your brush with kidney disease will guide people with hypertension, diabetes, urinary infection, or hematuria and proteinuria. Possibly you will save them from reaching end-stage renal disease (ESRD).
3. People may ignore you and call you names. You may be scoffed at, but later if your warning was unheeded and they face a similar situation, they will have only their egos to blame.

4. Be your own master in health matters. Search, find information, and talk to people at the clinic or dialysis center. You will learn to accept your situation. Maybe yours will be better compared to others'.

Need for Support

A person who is already facing a health challenge should make use of common sense to catch himself or herself before plunging into depression. Once this low mental state sets in, help from counselors must be considered seriously to decrease impact of two major conditions—chronic kidney disease and depression—that could lead to a very grave situation.

Counseling is help given by qualified people who know how to help people retrace their steps and find the road to survival. However qualified or experienced the counselor may be, you may wish to choose someone who understands you well.

Please do some research before you sign up for counseling. Your friends or physician could guide you in this matter.

Being physically and mentally fit to receive your treatment is important.

Remember this always so you don't miss your opportunity:

All of us are important to our families.
We have to keep our intrinsic values one notch higher—
Keep learning skills, try to work and earn, and
Smile through life.
No one cares for a loser.
A winner is not one great successful person.
It is one who will stand head held high,
Not in pride but in humility.
CKD is a great teacher of humility,
Humility brings you honor and, with it, bountiful joy!
See that you keep the fire of love burning,
Being your kind self.

Diet for Kidney Disease and Life

Be watchful of what you eat based on what you must eat. That's the only way to live with kidney disease. There's no other way. Talk to your doctor and dietician. Their guidance will be of great help. Make your small sacrifices. Forgo or limit what is not to be eaten. It is better to measure the permissible portion and eat within the limits suggested by your doctor/dietician. Learn to break your dietary rules on a rare day, but go back to doing what provides you with good health and comfort. CKD is no joke.

Learn to live with knowledge of all the essentials.

Exercise

Like diet, exercise is critical for managing all stages of kidney disease. You may discuss with your doctor what is best suited for your condition. Make a regular schedule for exercise. Thereafter, try to keep to the schedule.

THE RIDE BEYOND REJECTION

Vasundhara Raghavan

The rhythm of life is determined by many celestial influences, even as our universe makes its own moves or as the waves of the sea change their motion.

Who gets to keep their kidney and who loses their kidney is a matter decided by a throw of the dice.

Many people live with their valuable kidney for twenty, thirty, forty, or even fifty years. The dice simply did not select their kidney. Try to tell the aggrieved about this elusive game of dice. It will make sense even if some are more stubborn about their rights. In time, the understanding will surface that not everyone was meant to be a star.

That said, note that it is very, very difficult to understand the why of losing a kidney and to accept it gracefully. To attain a mastery of the philosophy of chance, one has some swallowing to do—of pride and of overwhelming emotion—while letting tears flow freely without any inhibition. The anger, the desperateness, is an integral part of the game. So time is needed for the mind to leave the throne and let the heart lead so that kneeling meekly in submission of the superior power is possible.

Life can then be picked up piece by piece. Surely no one wants to let anyone else tread on scattered pieces of their own self-esteem.

FACING KIDNEY FAILURE

Vasundhara Raghavan

Kidney transplants definitely rank higher than dialysis as successful treatment, but in spite of many medical advances, there's a chance of a graft failure.

Research has shown that people who receive live donor transplants have better survival rates.

Figure 3. Survival rates for kidney transplants

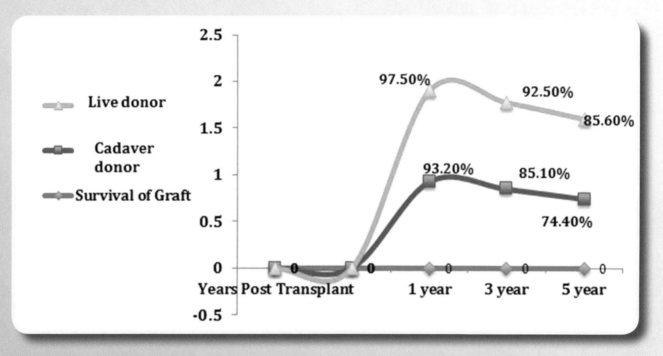

Data taken from Kidney Kaplan-Meier Survival Rates for transplants performed 2008–2015. Based on OPTN data as of October 20, 2017. Organ Procurement and Transplantation Network, USA. Table made by Vasundhara Raghavan.

Whether live donor or cadaver transplants, many transplants do fail for several reasons, as follows.

- Blood clot

If the blood vessels going to the transplanted kidney develop clots during the surgery, there is every likelihood that the kidney won't receive enough blood supply.

- Infections in the kidney

These can cause serious complications unless identified and treated early.

- Deep-rooted problems in the kidney

In some cases, though doctors have recommended the organ for transplant, there could be inherent deep-rooted problems in the kidney that could surface after the transplant. Some of these are treatable, while some could create a problem.

Early rejections must be promptly attended. At some point, the patient's proactive attention to his or her own health care can play a huge role in managing the kidney. The following are things the kidney transplant patient should do:

o   Be alert to catch signs of infections—cold, cough, fever—and take steps to communicate with and meet the doctor.
o   Be compliant on medications and water intake. Understanding the concept of a kidney transplant and the role of the immunosuppressant is extremely important. The medications suppress the immune system so the body does not attack the kidney. These medications are scheduled, so one must be conscious of the timing and take them every day to stay ahead in the "graft survival game."
o   Take simple precautions against infections.

Acute rejections can be managed with treatments. Though more common in the first few months, an acute rejection could happen at any time.

A chronic rejection means that the kidney is beyond recovery. The kidney is not accepted by the body and is a long-term problem. The kidney will give up in time.

Some medicines have a tendency to create a problem for the kidney. These could lead to kidney damage.

In some instances, fluid gets collected around the kidney. If this is not treated in time, it damages the kidney.

Also, there may be a recurrence of the earlier disease. Some diseases that cause kidney failure could reoccur.

Most often the transplant failure is not the result of negligence on the part of the kidney recipient. However, considering how difficult it is to get a transplant, the person receiving the transplant must make it a point to do the following things:

-   Communicate with the nephrologist about small or big issues experienced.
-   Ask for a change in medication if the side effects of certain medicines are severe.
-   Be always in control of one's health.

Rejection Makes Another Life Change

A person who receives the notice "Your graft has failed!" has to reckon with many aspects of life. However gently this news is delivered, the person's situation cannot be changed. When choosing to undergo transplant, the person is briefed on the survival rates of grafts while subtly being provided with the cons of a transplant. But reality is what determines the future.

The aftermath of a rejection awakens new perceptions of the future. What occurs is as follows:

- Shock – How can this be happening?
- Hurt and disappointment because the kidney failed, no matter if it lasted for five, ten, or twenty years.
- Fear. The fact that life went in reverse gear means the person must go back to dialysis. This gives rise to a great feeling of insecurity.
- Acceptance that dialysis needs to be started. Though most people receive a transplant after undergoing some dialysis treatments, once they experience a transplant, they need lots of encouragement to go back on dialysis.
- Sadness and frustration about having to again start the registration process for a transplant, if a second transplant is possible for the person.
- A feeling of abandonment. During the period that the kidney lasted, people who were once strong supporters the kidney patient moved on in life. A new loneliness envelopes the person at this point. He or she needs to be showered with love, assurance, and understanding. His or her file with the transplant team is inactive and they need to find new health support. If the rejection happens with ninety days of transplant, the transplant team may request that the person be given his or her initial wait time back.
- Relief. This is experienced by people whose transplant was a very traumatic experience. They may have faced many serious complications, handled many treatments, and endured side effects and multiple hospitalizations. In such a situation, it may seem better to be on dialysis.

Apart from the emotional outbursts, in the first few months there is a need to relearn many aspects of the disease that the person learned when his or her kidney disease was first detected. This is a great challenge. Following are things that need to be done:

- making dietary modifications for hemodialysis
- getting a fistula in place
- adapting to the rules of the "water game"

    o dialysis requires water restriction—two liters of fluid split across two days
    o post-transplant – consuming three to five liters of water each day (as advised by your transplant physician/nephrologist)
    o going back on dialysis – consuming two liters of fluid over two days

Though dietary changes are also a big issue to contend with, this swing in water consumption is most dramatic. In hot climates particularly, water restriction is very difficult. Lots of adjustments are needed to be healthy on dialysis, both emotionally and physically.

Good support from family, friends, and the community will steer the person to rise above the constraints and get registered for a transplant or look for another live donor. It is tough, but not impossible.

It is important for the person whose graft has stopped working to realize how important it is to be alive. Shifting focus onto other aspects of health care and looking for alternate dialysis treatments may help the person surviving with great positivity.

GLOSSARY OF TECHNICAL TERMS

access: Access is created for entering the bloodstream so that dialysis can be done. In the case of hemodialysis, a fistula acts as the access.

acute coronary syndrome: It involves chest pain and other symptoms, when the heart does not get enough blood.

acute kidney injury (AKI): A form of acute kidney failure, AKI is a sudden decline in kidney function. This happens most often as the result of the toxicity of certain medicines (e.g., painkillers and antibiotics); a drop in blood flow caused by severe infections such as sepsis; dehydration; and urethra blockage. It will lead to a buildup of waste products and create imbalance in electrolytes and body fluids. AKI requires treatment through acute dialysis and is recognized to be associated with greater risk of short-term and long-term death and adverse kidney outcomes.

albumin: A protein made by the liver, albumin is found in blood plasma, serum, muscle, the whites of eggs, milk, and other animal substances. A test of blood and urine is done for measuring protein in the blood and urine.

albuminuria/proteinuria: Presence of high albumin or protein in the urine is a sign of some damage to the kidneys. Proteinuria could be the result of long-term hyperglycemia (high blood sugar levels) of hypertension (high blood pressure).

anemia: If a person feels weak, breathless, and less energetic, it may be indicative of being anemic. When blood has a shortage of red cells, anemia occurs. For improvement, iron and erythropoietin will be needed.

angiotensin-converting enzyme inhibitors: Also known as ACE inhibitors, these are medications for the heart that help widen or dilate the blood vessels to improve the amount of blood the heart pumps and thereby lower blood pressure. By increasing blood flow, ACE inhibitors help to decrease the amount of work the heart has to do. Well-controlled blood pressure by some ACE inhibitors has enabled slow progression of kidney damage in many people with type 2 diabetes.

artery: A blood vessel that carries blood from the heart to the rest of the body.

bladder: From the kidney, the urine goes into the organ known as the bladder, before being released from the body.

blood cells: The blood is made up of microscopic cells that are known as blood cells. Blood cells consist of red and white cells and platelets.

blood group: Our blood can be classified into four main groups: A, B, AB, and O. The classification system is based on hereditary conditions dictating the availability of certain antigens in the cells. Generally blood and organ donations are based on the match of blood group between the donor and recipient.

blood pressure: When the blood passes through the arteries, it exerts a certain level of pressure against their walls. This pressure is measured as blood pressure. Blood pressure is an important determinant for many surgeries and indicates the health condition of a person.

- Normal blood pressure is 120/80 millimeters of mercury (mm Hg) or less.
- Prehypertension is between 120/80 mm Hg and 139/89 mm Hg.
- High blood pressure is more than 140/90 mm Hg.
- If you are over age sixty-five, blood pressure up to 150/90 mm Hg can be considered normal

body mass index (BMI): An individual's body mass (weight) by his or her height squared. It is a measurement of body fat.

bone marrow: In some bones, such as hip and thigh bones, there is a soft tissue in the hollow interior portion that is known as bone marrow. New blood cells get created here.

cadaveric transplant: This is a transplant surgery done with a kidney or other organ removed from a person who is brain-dead or has died in an accident.

calcium: This is a mineral salt that strengthens the bones.

catheter: A catheter is a flexible plastic tube that is inserted when access to the body's interior is needed.

cardiovascular: This relates to the heart and the blood vessels involved in blood circulation.

cholesterol: This is a measure of the level of fat in the bloodstream. There is a risk of having heart disease or stroke if the blood shows a high cholesterol value. Though high cholesterol is dangerous, the levels can be reduced with diet and drugs.

creatinine: When muscles are used, a waste substance known as creatinine is produced. A blood test is used to measure creatinine, and this measurement indicates whether or not the kidney is functioning normally.

The normal values for creatinine are 0.6–1.2 milligrams per deciliter (mg/dL).

crossmatch: The crossmatch is different from tissue type or blood group match. Crossmatch is a blood test to check for the existence of any antibodies. Antibodies normally help the body fight infection and would react with the donor kidney. High levels of antibodies may lead to rejection, even if it is a good tissue-type match.

Crossmatch is done by mixing a sample of the recipient's blood with cells from the donor. If the recipient's blood starts attacking the donor cells, there is the likelihood that the kidney will be rejected.

dehydration: The body is dehydrated when there is insufficient water in the body for its proper functioning.

diabetes: When high levels of glucose are found in the blood and urine, a condition popularly known as diabetes is said to be the problem. This happens because of poor functioning of the pancreas. The world over, people with diabetes are at high risk for kidney failure.

diabetic nephropathy: Kidney disease that results from diabetes, diabetic nephropathy is the number one cause of kidney failure. Almost one-third of people with diabetes develop diabetic nephropathy at some point unless there is strict control of diabetes through medications.

dialysis: The process of removing the waste products and excess water from the blood when the kidneys cease to perform this function properly is known as dialysis.

dialyzer: A dialysis machine has a filtering unit known as a dialyzer, which removes waste products and excess water from the blood.

dietary acid load (DAL): The body's metabolism produces acids and bases of varying levels based on food consumed. The difference between the acids and bases is called the dietary acid load (DAL) or, formally, net endogenous acid production (NEAP). These acids must be buffered or excreted by the body through respiration or urination in order to maintain an acid–base balance.

diuretic drugs: Medicines administered to increase urine outputs are called diuretics.

donor: A person who donates an organ, blood, or tissue to another person is known as a donor.

dry weight: The body weight after dialysis is called a dry weight. The weight is without excess fluid in the lungs or in the tissues.

dyslipidemia: This condition is marked by abnormal concentrations of lipids or lipoproteins such as cholesterol in the blood.

dysrhythmia: This is an abnormal rhythm, especially a disordered rhythm exhibited in a record of electrical activity of the brain or heart.

edema: This is an abnormal accumulation of water in the body. If the water is accumulated in the lungs, it is called pulmonary edema.

end-stage renal disease (ESRD): When the kidney loses all its functions and reaches the final stage of irreversible loss, it has reached ESRD. Such result may be expected from diabetes, chronic hypertension, or glomerulonephritis.

epidemiology: The study of the distribution and determinants of health-related states or events in specified populations, and the application of this study to control health problems.

erythropoietin (EPO): When the kidney functions properly, this is a hormone that it produces, along with several others. This hormone stimulates the bone marrow to produce red blood cells. But when the kidney fails, the person may become anemic if lower levels of red blood cells get produced. In such a situation, EPO injections may be given to perform the hormone's function.

expanded criteria donor (ECD): Apart from ideal candidates for organ donation, now people not considered to be ideal or standard are being evaluated as a possible donors. With these criteria, donors who may be included are people of advanced ages, people who have been previous infected with hepatitis B or hepatitis C, people with hypertension or diabetes mellitus, people who have abnormal donor organ function, or a person whose heart is no longer beating (i.e., deceased).

fistula: In order to provide access to the bloodstream for hemodialysis, a vein may be enlarged surgically. This access is called a fistula.

fluid overload: This is excess water in the body caused by excess consumption of water or not being able to pass enough urine.

glomerular filtration rate (GFR): Glomerular filtration is the process by which the kidneys filter the blood, removing excess wastes and fluids. To determine the level of the kidney's functioning a GFR is calculated that shows how well the blood is filtered by the kidneys. That is one way to measure remaining kidney function. GFR is usually an estimate, so it is eGFR arrived at by using a mathematical formula that is based on a person's size, age, sex, and race to compare serum creatinine levels.

GFR: How to Interpret It

Stage	What this means	GFR level
At increased risk	Kidneys are at risk due to diabetes, high blood pressure, family history, old age, and/or ethnic group	More than 90
1	Some damage with normal kidney function	90 or above
2	Damage with mild loss of kidney function	89 to 60
3a	Mild to moderate loss of kidney function	59 to 44
3b	Moderate to severe loss of kidney function	44 to 30
4	Very severe loss of kidney function	29 to 15
5	Kidney failure	Less than 15

The GFR number tells you at what level of kidney function remains.
Your doctor will tell you the stage of kidney disease.
GFR goes down with the progression of kidney disease.

Information source: National Kidney Foundation

glucose: A sugar found in the blood that is used by cells to produce energy.

glycemia: The presence of glucose in the blood.

glycemic control: For people with diabetes, it is important to have a glycemic control, which means to have blood sugar at acceptable levels over a prolonged period, usually measured by hemoglobin A1c or fasting blood glucose.

hemodialysis (HD): A more popular form of dialysis for blood purification. The blood is cleaned outside the body by a dialysis machine, a process that takes between three and four hours to finish.

hemoglobin: The red blood cells have hemoglobin, which carries oxygen to all parts of the body.

hemoglobin A1c test: This test, also called HbA1c, glycated hemoglobin test, or glycohemoglobin, will determine how well diabetes is being controlled. HbA1c gives an average of blood glucose control over a six- to twelve-week period, which, along with periodic home blood glucose monitoring, is useful to appropriately treat diabetes.

ideal body weight: An ideal body weight is determined based on the age, sex, and height of the person. This is the expected range for people falling within that group.

immune system: Everybody has an immune system that protects the body from infections and foreign bodies. In the case of a person who has had a transplant, the system is suppressed by medication so that it does not reject the foreign organ. The immune system therefore works less effectively.

immunosuppressant drugs: These are drugs prescribed to transplant patients to make the immune system less effective so that it does not fight the foreign body, which is the transplanted kidney or other organ. Immunosuppressant drugs are required to protect the kidney from being rejected.

macroalbuminuria: Albuminuria is defined as a relatively high rate of urinary excretion of albumin, which could be greater than 300 milligrams per twenty-four-hour period.

malnutrition: This condition occurs because of weight loss due to lower consumption of food providing protein and energy.

nasogastric tube: This is normally called the NG tube. It is made of a flexible material such as rubber or plastic. The tube, used to put substances, including nutrients, into the stomach, is inserted through the nose and then through the esophagus into the stomach when a patient is unable to eat or drink by mouth.

Sometimes the tube is used to remove contents from the stomach, including air, small solid objects, fluid, and toxic substances that cannot be removed normally through the stool.

nephritis: This is an inflammation of the kidneys.

nephron: The kidney is made up of many small units called nephrons, which do the filtering and balance fluid in the body.

omentum: The omentum hangs like a curtain from the bottom of the stomach, right in front of the intestines. It is like a sheet of fatty tissue that stores body fat, and it grows as more fat is accumulated. It contains germ-fighting cells that can migrate to the abdomen and helps to seal it off. The omentum therefore protects the abdomen from infections. For the surgeon the omentum acts as a handy tool—something like biological duct tape. Portions of the omentum may be used as a graft in cut areas to heal them. The omentum can also be a source of problems. When its blood supply is interrupted, there are symptoms of severe pain and tenderness that can wrongly be diagnosed as appendicitis. Another aspect is that when it is enlarged due to high fat storage, it results in a protruding belly, and the person does not look very pleasing.

peritoneal cavity: This is the area in the abdomen where the stomach, liver, and bowels are found.

peritoneal dialysis (PD): This form of dialysis uses the peritoneum as a filter. The blood is cleaned inside the person's body, not externally, as in hemodialysis. PD is a home dialysis program.

peritoneum: This is a natural membrane lining the walls of the abdomen.

phosphate: An important substance involved with calcium that accumulates when the kidneys fail.

phosphate binders: In order to avoid the buildup of phosphate in the blood, phosphate binders are prescribed. They absorb excess phosphorus in the blood.

platelets: These are a type of blood cell that helps in clotting blood.

polycystic kidney disease: This kidney disease is hereditary and occurs because of a problem with kidney development. The kidneys get enlarged and are full of sacs filled with fluid, which are known as cysts. This disease sometimes leads to kidney failure.

potassium: This mineral is normally present in the blood, but it has to be maintained at a particular level. Higher or lower levels may cause heart problems.

protein: This is essential for muscle formation, and the breakdown products are filtered by the kidney. Meat, fish, dairy products, and nuts are rich in protein.

proteinuria: The presence of excess protein in the urine.

pulmonary edema: When the lungs get filled with fluid, the resulting condition is known as pulmonary edema. It results in breathlessness, especially when lying down flat and exercising.

pyelonephritis: This is a painless inflammation caused by repeated infections, drugs, or other factors. It occurs in the part of the kidney that is in between the filtering units.

recipient: A person who receives an organ for transplant from a donor.

rejection: The immune system fights infection and foreign bodies. In the case of a transplant, the organ transplanted is in fact a foreign body. The immune system may attack the organ, leading to rejection.

renal: It is the term used for kidneys. A renal failure means a failure of the kidneys.

restless legs syndrome (RLS): This neurological disorder causes an individual to experience an uncomfortable sensation in his or her legs, leading to an urge to move them. Symptoms occur most often at night, as lying down tends to activate the symptoms. The disorder affects both males and females, with a twice as high an incidence in females. With age this syndrome gets worse.

satellite hemodialysis unit: A unit that is located away from the main hospital renal unit and provides hemodialysis is known as a satellite unit.

semipermeable: A membrane that allows some substances to pass through it is called semipermeable.

serum: The fluid portion of the blood obtained after removal of the fibrin clot and blood cells, distinguished from the plasma in circulating blood.

serum creatinine: A product of creatinine phosphate that is filtered from the blood by the kidneys. Serum creatinine levels rise with decreased renal function.

Tenckhoff catheter: In peritoneal dialysis, the catheter that allows access for the dialysis fluid to flow in and out from the peritoneal cavity, but that is capped off when not in use, is known as a Tenckhoff catheter.

tissue type: A blood test called a tissue type test is conducted to measure the antigens on the surface of the body and its cells.

transplant: This surgery is done to plant a new organ, which is donated by someone, into a patient who needs it for survival.

ultrafiltration: This process removes excess water from the blood.

underdialysis: This happens when dialysis treatment is not sufficient to remove all the water and waste products that are in excess.

urea: This is one of the main waste products that build up in the blood. In addition to creatinine levels, the levels of urea in the blood are indicative of how the kidneys are functioning.

ureters: Urine is carried from the kidneys to the bladder through tubes called ureters.

urethra: The tube that carries urine from the bladder outside the body is called the urethra.

urine: This is the fluid produced by the kidneys. It is composed of excess water and the toxic waste products that come from food and are not required by the body.

urine protein-to-creatinine ratio (UPCR): This is the ratio of urinary protein to creatinine used to quantify the amount of protein being excreted through urine and used to calculate proteinuria.

veins: Blood vessels that carry dark-red-colored blood are veins. They bring impure blood from different parts of the body to the heart for purification. They have less oxygen and are thinner than arteries.

SOURCES

Listed below are some materials we referenced during the process of writing *Who Lives, Who Dies with Kidney Disease*. They helped in our understanding, and they provide readers with information in simple layperson's language.

American Heart Association – www.heart.org/HEARTORG
American Kidney Fund – www.kidneyfund.org
American Urology Association – www.auanet.org
Astellas Transplant – www.transplantexperience.com
Cedar-Sinai Medical Center – www.csmc.edu
Davita – www.davita.com
eMedicineHealth – www.emedicinehealth.com
Healthcommunities.com – www.healthcommunities.com
The Kidney Foundation of Canada – www.kidney.ca
Kidney School – www.kidneyschool.org
Mayo Clinic – www.mayoclinic.com
MedlinePlus Medical Encyclopedia – www.nlm.nih.gov/medlineplus/encyclopedia.html
MedicineNet.com – www.medicinenet.com
Merriam-Webster Online Dictionary – www.merriam-webster.com
National Kidney Foundation, India – www.nkfi.in
National Kidney Foundation, Southern California – www.kidney.org
National Kidney Foundation, United States – www.kidney.org
National Kidney and Urological Diseases Information Clearinghouse – kidney.niddk.nih.gov/kudiseases
Nephrology Channel – www.nephrologychannel.com
Texas Pediatric Surgical Associates – www.pedisurg.com
University of Iowa Hospitals and Clinics – www.uihealthcare.com
University of Pennsylvania Health System – www.pennmedicine.org
WebMD – https://www.webmd.com/

Acharya, V. N. "Status of Renal Transplant in India," *Journal of Postgraduate Medicine* 40, no. 1 (1994): 158–61. http://www.jpgmonline.com.

Faris, Michie Hall, *When Your Kidneys Fail*. Southern California: National Kidney Foundation, 1994.

Garovoy, Marvin R., and Ronald D. Guttmann. *Renal Transplantation*. New York: Churchill Livingstone, 1986.

Stein, Andy, and Janet Wild. *Kidney Dialysis and Transplants*. London: Class Publishing, 2002.

OUR GRATITUDE

In the process of writing *Who Lives, Who Dies with Kidney Disease,* **we met and got closely** connected with people who had a singular goal and purpose: to survive the insurmountable chronic kidney disease.

Conscious of how inspiration is always needed in huge doses, they agreed to impart their life experiences to encourage many people to find their individual treatment goals.

We are forever grateful for this community of people who came together to add value to *Who Lives, Who Dies with Kidney Disease.*

Dr. Mohammad Akmal
Vasundhara Raghavan

Kidney disease was never your choice.

It just happened.

Love yourself.
Fight to survive.

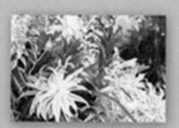

19-02-2017

Printed in the United States
By Bookmasters